HEALING WITH
MEDICAL
MARIJUANA

GETTING BEYOND THE
SMOKE AND MIRRORS

D1086905

HEALING WITH MEDICAL MARIJUANA

GETTING BEYOND THE SMOKE AND MIRRORS

Dr. Mark Sircus

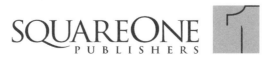

SQUAREONE
PUBLISHERS

The information and advice contained in this book are based upon the research and the personal and professional experiences of the authors. They are not intended as a substitute for consulting with a health care professional. The publisher and author are not responsible for any adverse effects or consequences resulting from the use of any of the suggestions, preparations, or procedures discussed in this book. All matters pertaining to your physical health should be supervised by a health care professional. It is a sign of wisdom, not cowardice, to seek a second or third opinion.

EDITOR: Erica Shur
COVER DESIGNER: Jeannie Tudor
TYPESETTER: Gary A. Rosenberg

Square One Publishers
115 Herricks Road
Garden City Park, NY 11040
(516) 535-2010 • (877) 900-BOOK
www.squareonepublishers.com

Library of Congress Cataloging-in-Publication Data

Names: Sircus, Mark, author.
Title: Healing with medical marijuana : getting beyond the smoke and mirrors / Dr. Mark Sircus.
Description: Garden City Park, NY : Square One Publishers, [2017] | Includes bibliographical references and index.
Identifiers: LCCN 2016050925 | ISBN 9780757004414 (pb)
ISBN 9780757054419 (eb)
Subjects: LCSH: Marijuana—Health aspects. | Marijuana—Therapeutic use.
Classification: LCC RM666.C266 S57 2016 | DDC 615.3/2345—dc23
LC record available at https://lccn.loc.gov/2016050925

Printed in the United States of America

10   9   8   7   6   5   4   3   2   1

Contents

Preface

There is a hurricane wind of change around the subject of drugs, especially marijuana in recent years, yet in July of 2016 the U.S. government announced that marijuana would continue to be classified as a Schedule 1 drug, meaning it has a high potential for abuse even though there is a rising tide of humanitarianism screaming for full legalization. Then in August, a federal court ruled that the Department of Justice could not spend money to prosecute people who violate federal drug laws but comply with state medical marijuana laws.

The ruling prevents federal law enforcement from prosecution of anyone who obeys a state's medical marijuana laws yet congress could change that. The "war on drugs" is one of the most irrational and destructive public policy failures in American history that has police officers arresting more than 1.2 million people a year in the United States on charges of illegal drug possession.

More Americans are using marijuana, and fewer people think that regularly doing so is harmful. A study published in *The Lancet Psychiatry* shows that from 2002 to 2014, the number of American adults who used marijuana in the last year increased by 10 million and the number of people who used it daily increased by more than four million. More adults also started using marijuana for the first time. Yet there was not an increase in reported marijuana abuse or dependence. The researchers observed a drop—50 percent to 33 percent—in the number of people who thought that smoking marijuana once or twice a week was harmful.

In medical-marijuana states, the average doctor prescribed 265 fewer doses of antidepressants each year, 486 fewer doses of seizure medication, 541 fewer antinausea doses and 562 fewer doses of anti-anxiety medication. However, most strikingly, the typical physician in a medical-marijuana state prescribed 1,826 fewer doses of painkillers in a given year. Now only a few years later half of the states and Washington, D.C. have legalized medical marijuana to treat certain health problems, including painful nerve conditions and depression. It is my hope that this book will be helpful in offering medical options.

The greatest story to tell about marijuana is that it has an almost unlimited ability to calm human suffering, and because of this people are turning to medical marijuana as a preferred treatment to their pain and depression. There is more than enough evidence to suggest that marijuana could help people with anxiety and singlehandedly help end the opioid epidemic that is killing increasing amounts of people.

There are now unlimited anecdotal patient reports, increasing numbers of legitimate clinical case studies, and large amounts of preclinical studies that all indicate tumor-fighting activities of cannabinoids. Medical marijuana in concentrated form is a natural form of chemotherapy—it cures cancer! It might not cure everyone's cancer, and it does not address every cause—for that one needs a full cancer protocol. However, no cancer patient should do without it and that importantly includes the children who have cancer.

Medical scientists are studying whether marijuana can stave off Alzheimer's disease or even mitigate brain damage from stroke or concussions. A 2014 study suggested a compound in marijuana could slow the production of proteins that accumulate when a person has Alzheimer's. Cannabis helps cancer and HIV patients and others who suffer from the most severe cases of chronic pain.

The wind has changed in terms of marijuana and its ancient use as a helpmate to humans. The amount of healing benefits that come along with the various applications of marijuana is undeniable. The hope is that sometime in the near future, there will be widespread access to not only hemp health products but marijuana for medical and recreational purposes as well.

No matter how much good there is to be found in the marijuana plant there will always be people who are against its legalization. Though it is natural and generally safe, it seems threatening to people who do not use it. It was just stated by The Christian Science Monitor that there are more retail marijuana stores in Colorado than McDonalds and that there is a backlash to legalization in that state. However, there is little that is wholesome about McDonalds, its food is not healthy and many have made a case for its danger. A steady diet of fast food will make one sick quite quickly, but that is not the case with marijuana. One can go decades smoking marijuana without much of a problem but as you will read in this book is that it is not without its own toxicity, no matter how mild that might be.

Introduction

There is a quiet revolution occurring in this country. State by state, people are being given the right to use medical marijuana as a legitimate treatment against a wide variety of health disorders. More and more doctors are now prescribing the various forms of medical marijuana to help their patient. However, this revolution is not without its critics. They argue that there isn't any proof that it works; they say that its production is unregulated; and they even liken it to the use of a highly-addictive narcotic. The problem with their arguments is that they are untrue. Dig a little deeper into these opposition groups and you discover that many them are being funded by large private interests that feel threatened by the introduction of a safer alternative to many drugs.

As you will read, the fact is that there many scientifically-conducted studies that show the use of medical marijuana works. Unfortunately, because of a lack of Federal funding, the majority of these studies are conducted outside the United States. And while this seems to be a bone of contention from the opposition, that doesn't make the studies any less legitimate. The studies that have been carried out over the year are conducted by top researchers in their fields and at state-of-the-art hospitals and laboratories. Their findings have been published in peer-reviewed medical journals that provide the very evidence that medical marijuana is effective.

MY APPROACH

Based on the scientific work of so many others, I have put together this book to help you first understand the basics behind the use of these marijuana compounds and then how to appropriately use them. Although it is principally about medical marijuana, it is also a book on general medicine or what I call Natural Allopathic Medicine. As you will see, I have developed a comprehensive protocol around cannabinoid medicine where medical marijuana can be prescribed (or simply just taken) in combination with certain other substances (like magnesium oil) to amplify its effectiveness across a broad spectrum of disorders.

Magnesium chloride and cannabinoids blend together magnificently in harmony, and I like to think of them as the "Batman and Robin" of the medical world. Cannabinoid medicine is one strong part of the universal protocol I have created. This book is dominated by the presentation of cannabinoid medicine, but it is in the context of what could someday be known as the heavyweight gang of four medicinals that should be used together for best medical results.

It explains how my Natural Allopathic Medical approach combines cannabinoid medicine with magnesium medicine and then with pH and iodine medicine. Hopefully, *Healing With Medical Marijuana* makes it clear how the safest and least expensive medicines can outperform most pharmaceuticals by an extremely wide margin. As a medicine, marijuana is without equal carrying less danger than aspirin or any other pharmaceutical on the market. One can use it safely for decades and not suffer anything near the damage of using alcohol or most pharmaceuticals. Life is difficult enough on our planet, and it is about to get even more difficult. Marijuana can help us endure.

WHAT'S IN THIS BOOK

Healing With Medical Marijuana is divided into two parts. Part 1 is divided into 8 chapters, and in those chapters you will learn the fundamental science behind the use of medical marijuana. In Chapter 1 you will discover what makes up the cannabis herb and its benefits as a therapeutic drug. In the next three chapters you will be provided with material explaining why medical marijuana can be considered an essential medicine; its safety for adults as well as children; and how it is being used as a pediatric medicine. Although there are no existing fixed dosages for medical marijuana, Chapter 5 and 6 provides safe therapeutic dosages and possible delivery systems. The importance of hemp oil as a therapeutic drug is discussed in Chapter 7 as well as instructions for home production of hemp oil, and Chapter 8 takes you through the laws and the campaign against medical marijuana through the years. There are numerous quotes included in the text that I hope you will find meaningful. Please note that any quotes without attribution are mine.

Part 2 acts as a guide, providing you with a listing of health conditions, their symptoms, and their triggers. You will learn how one will benefit from using medical marijuana to treat the disorder, the conventional medicine usually recommended and their side effects, and how to use medical marijuana as a treatment for the diseases or health disorders.

I am a great proponent of medical marijuana as well as its use for relaxation, recreation, and de-stressing. However that does not mean it is a perfect substance. It does have its downsides. For people with breathing disorders, such as COPD, they should never smoke marijuana. In addition, some marijuana leaves contain cadmium contaminations as well as fungal contaminations which can be very harmful. Care must always be taken with any medicinal. As with any medicine there are warnings, precautions and contraindications. To this end, I have included important information on such precautions as well as a discussion of addiction.

WE HAVE A CHOICE

As you read this book, consider the following: We have become victimized by the pharmaceutical industry. In many cases, all you have to do is pay attention to any drug advertisement you hear on TV. It usually ends with the long citation of warnings, in many cases ending with "unexpected deaths have been reported." Then there is the practice of superficially jacked up pricing making some drugs almost impossible to buy a needed drug—not because it cost more to produce, but rather to increase the company's bottom line.

It is my hope that *Heal With Medical Marijuana* can offer you a sane and safer alternative—a product created by nature. The most important thing to remember as you read this book is the more you know, the better decisions you can make about your health and the ones you love.

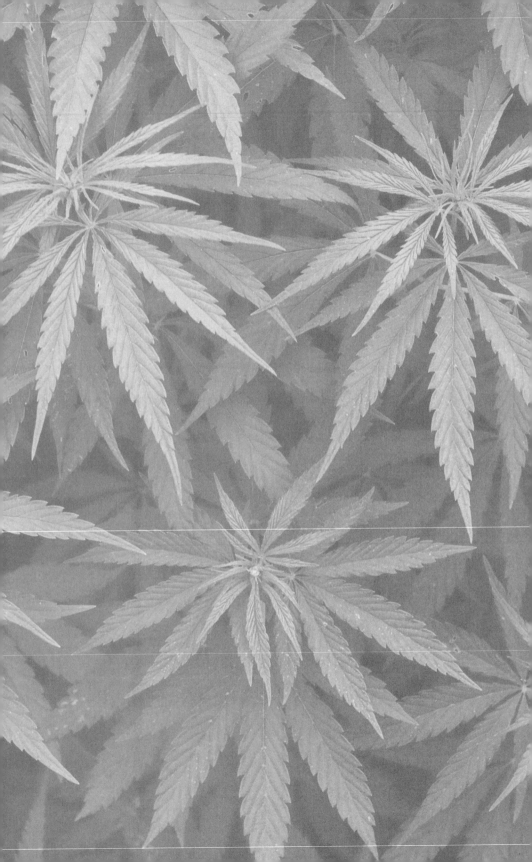

PART I

THE BASICS
Using Nature's Medicine to Heal

1.

Cannabis—
The Holy Herb

Marijuana is a "holy herb" and it deserves the attention of humanity. Marijuana is a colloquial term used to refer to the dried flowers of the female cannabis sativa and cannabis indica plants. Marijuana, or cannabis, as it is more appropriately called, has been part of humanity's medicine chest for almost as long as history has been recorded.

In 1992 Richard Evans Schultes and Albert Hoffman published *Plants of the Gods—Their Sacred, Healing and Hallucinogenic Powers*. In it they say that, "Tradition in India maintains that the gods sent man the hemp plant so that he might attain delight, courage, and have heightened sexual desires. The Indian vadas sang of Cannabis as one of the divine nectars, able to give man anything from good health and long life to visions of the gods. If taken over a long term, it makes one communicate with spirits and lightens one's body.

A Taoist priest wrote in the fifth century B.C. that Cannabis was employed by "necromancers, in combination with Ginseng, to set forward time and reveal future events. It was in ancient India that this 'gift of the gods' founded excessive use in folk medicine. It was believed to quicken the mind, prolong life, improve judgment, lower fevers, induce sleep, and cure dysentery. Because of its psychoactive properties it was more highly valued than medicines with only physical activity. Several systems of Indian medicine esteemed cannabis. It was in the Himalayas of India and the Tibetan plateau that cannabis preparations assumed their greatest hallucinogenic importance in religious contexts. The Tibetans considered cannabis sacred. A Mahayana Buddhist tradition maintains that during the six steps of asceticism leading to his enlightenment, Buddha lived on one hemp seed a day."

FOR THERAPEUTIC USE

Cannabis was formally introduced to the United States Pharmacopoeia (USP) in 1854, though written references regarding the plant's therapeutic use date back as far as 2800 B.C. By 1900, cannabis was the third leading active ingredient, behind alcohol and opiates, in patent medicines for sale in America.

Cannabis was a common ingredient in medications until 1937, when the plant was outlawed by the Marijuana Tax Act despite the objections of the American Medical Association. Possibly the best thing the AMA has done in its long history is to fight the removal of marijuana from the textbooks and lists of medicines in their pharmacopeia.

Chemistry of Cannabis

The chemistry of cannabis is quite complex. There are over 400 chemicals in marijuana, but only about 80 are unique to the cannabis plant and these are classified as cannabinoids. Among the most psychoactive of the cannabinoids is delta-9-tetrahydrocannabinol (THC), the active ingredient in the prescription medications dronabinol (Marinol), and naboline (Cesamet). Other major cannabinoids include cannabidiol (CBD) and cannabinol (CBN), both of which are non-psychoactive but possess distinct pharmacological effects.

Cannabinoid Receptors

Cannabinoids, when consumed by humans, bind to CB1 and CB2 cannabinoid receptors in the brain and body, causing euphoria and important pharmacological effects. These receptors are proteins that bind with cannabinoids. The synergy between these receptors and cannabinoids are known to provide protective effects against inflammation in the brain. THC that targets cannabinoid receptors CB1 and CB2 is similar in function to endocannabinoids, which are cannabinoids that are naturally produced in the body and activate these receptors.

The CB1 receptors have been found in the brain in areas that control the coordination of movement, emotions, memory, reduction of pain, reward systems, and reproduction, yet are almost absent in the brain stem (which affects our vital functions, such as breathing). While the CB1 receptors are primarily found in the central nervous system, CB2, discovered in 1993, are found primarily in the immune system, GI tract, liver, spleen, kidney, bones, heart, and peripheral nervous system. In fact, the CB2 receptor appears to be upregulated whenever there is tissue pathology.

Endocannabinoid System

The cannabinoid receptors, endocannabinoids and the related enzymes make up what is now called the endocannabinoid system and this system is essential in most if not all physiological systems. The endocannabinoid system is essential to life and it relates messages that affect how we relax, eat, and sleep.

The fact that we have receptors in our brains for the cannabinoids in marijuana, or what has been universally known through the ages as the hemp plant, speaks of a nutritional type of relationship. Our bodies are receptive to cannabinoids—incredibly so—so much so that it's a euphoric relationship. Cannabinoids fit in like keys into our cannabinoid system and our cells like it! Our body enjoys these keys so much that it is healed from them.

Cannabis as a Drug

Marijuana is a wonder drug! When pharmaceutical companies no longer deliver their drugs, when economies collapse into deep depressions, we will have to learn to take care of ourselves with marijuana, a medicine we can grow at home for little cost. Marijuana was given to us by Nature for many uses and can only be considered beneficial if one is at all concerned with safe medicine and health.

CBD has anti-inflammatory, anti-anxiety, anti-epileptic, sedative, and neuro-protective actions. It is also a potent anti-oxidant, protecting against chemical damage due to oxidation. Studies have suggested that CBD could protect against the development of diabetes, certain kinds of cancer, rheumatoid arthritis, brain and nerve damage due to stroke, alcoholism, nausea, inflammatory bowel disease, and Huntington's disease.

A cannabinoid derivative, dexanabinol (HU-211), could be the first neuroprotective agent to be approved for human use by the FDA. If it is successful it might become a "standard inclusion in the kit bag of every medic and ambulance", says neurosurgeon Nachshon Knoller from Israel.

Dexanabinol is a non-psychotropic derivative of a synthetic family of tetrahydrocannabinoid analogues. The drug has three independent mechanisms of action: it blocks glutamate-induced neurotoxicity; it scavenges both peroxy and hydroxy free radicals; and it inhibits the action of the inflammatory cytokine alpha-tumor necrosis factor. "The triple action stops the spread of the primary neuronal damage from the core of injury to the surrounding brain tissue, even after a single intravenous injection, up to six hours after the initial insult," says Raphael Mechoulam, Professor of Pharmacology, Hadassah Medical School, Jerusalem, Israel.

The results of a U.K. phase I clinical trial showing lack of adverse reactions to dexanabinol and results from earlier animal studies were presented on November 15, 1996 in Washington, DC, USA at the annual meeting of the Society of Neurotrauma. A phase II clinical study of dexanabinol started in Israel on November 9th, under the auspices of the American Brain Injury Consortium, in patients with severe head injury exhibiting abnormal computed tomography scans and requiring intracranial pressure monitoring.

The class of interneurons the researchers studied called "LTS cells" of the cerebral cortex, manufacture and release cannabinoids that bind to their own cannabinoid receptors and shut down their ability to signal other neurons. By shutting themselves off, the interneurons block their quieting action on the excitatory pyramidal cells—an effect that can last as long as 35 minutes, much longer than what had been seen with retrograde inhibition. Without the quieting effect, pyramidal cells signal more intensely, triggering a higher level of activity in circuits of the cortex.

Anti-inflammatory

Many doctors and books are talking about inflammation today but they fail to mention medical marijuana as a mighty muscleman in the anti-inflammation world. The newest, strongest and possibly greatest anti-inflammatory on the block, cannabidiol (CBD), is legal and now exists and is available in topical and oral forms. People who have used medical marijuana know this because it gives so much quick pain relief. Even oncologists prescribe marijuana for pain.

Natural Chemotherapy

Researchers at the University of Milan in Naples, Italy reported in the *Journal of Pharmacology and Experimental Therapeutics* that non-psychoactive compounds in marijuana inhibited the growth of glioma cells in a dose-dependent manner, and selectively targeted and killed malignant cells through apoptosis. "Non-psychoactive CBD (cannabidiol) produces a significant anti-tumor activity both *in vitro* and *in vivo*, thus suggesting a possible application of CBD as an antineoplastic agent."

Cannabinoids offer cancer patients a therapeutic option in the treatment of highly invasive cancers. The medical science is strongly in favor of hemp oil as a primary cancer therapy, not just in a supportive role to control the side effects of chemotherapy. Researchers at the California Pacific Medical Center Research Institute (CPMCRI) combined the non-psychoactive cannabis compound, cannabidiol (CBD), with Δ9-tetrahyrdocannabinol (9-THC), the primary psychoactive active ingredient in cannabis. They found the combination boosts the inhibitory effects of Δ9-THC on glioblastoma, the most common and aggressive form of brain tumor, and the cancer that claimed the life of Senator Ted Kennedy.

BENEFICIAL EFFECTS AND SAFETY

In general, what divides the chemicals and heavy metals found in pharmaceutical medicines from nutritional substances is that one has damaging side effects and can hurt or kill and the other makes the cells sing. We can take most nutritional substances in high dosages, even when they are concentrated.

But pharmaceutical drugs are killers and need to be used with extreme caution, something most doctors have forgotten about because they blindly trust drug companies, the FDA, and their teachers in medical school.

Marijuana is one of the most complicated broad-acting medicinal in existence on earth and can be used to provide improved medical treatment at a greatly reduced cost. In this book you will find a lot of surprising information and research that indicates that cannabinoids represent a Holy Grail for medicine. In its natural unprocessed form it can out-perform every other class of medicine in terms of safety and effectiveness, so doctors need to pay attention, and many are. The only other medicinal that runs neck-and-neck with cannabinoid medicine is magnesium medicine and you will *always* find me advocating taking the two together.

According to Dr. Lester Grinspoon, "A poll conducted by Medscape, a website directed at health care providers, cited that 76 percent of physicians and 89 percent of nurses said they thought marijuana should be available as a medicine. The dramatic change of view is the result of clinical experience. Doctors and nurses have seen that for many patients cannabis is more useful, less toxic, and less expensive than the conventional medicines prescribed for diverse syndromes and symptoms, including multiple sclerosis, Crohn's disease, migraine headaches, severe nausea and vomiting, convulsive disorders, the AIDS wasting syndrome, chronic pain, and many others."

CONCLUSION

In a toxic world the antioxidant effects of marijuana might make it a required medicinal for survival in the 21st century. However, even as marijuana becomes more popular, especially in medical and health circles, a campaign continues not only against users but also against researchers.

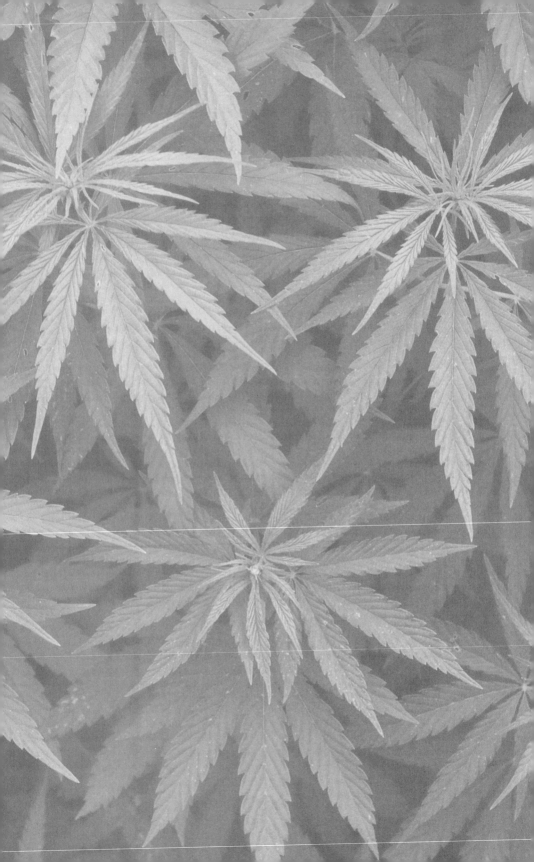

2.

The Essential Medicine

What is medical marijuana? Medical marijuana refers to using the whole unprocessed marijuana plant or its basic extracts to treat a disease or symptom. The Department of Justice ruled that marijuana has no medical value at all, and can't be used safely because of a high potential for abuse even when given under a doctor's supervision. However, scientific studies of the chemicals in marijuana, called cannabinoids, have led to medications that consist of cannabinoid chemicals and have been approved by the FDA.

Dr. Allan Frankel says, "As a short-term life-prolonging medicine and a long-term therapy for chronic conditions, medical cannabis is a miracle drug that is endorsed by countless doctors and nurses, as well as the patients whose lives are dramatically improved by its use." Marijuana as a medicine is a strong, safe, easy to use and extremely inexpensive if you grow it yourself as a weed in the backyard or living room. The pharmaceutical industry has nothing pharmacologically equal to cannabinoids.

Advocates of medical cannabis have used the CBD and THC found in cannabis for a variety of illnesses throughout history. Right now, there are hundreds of thousands of patients using marijuana safely, effectively—and under a doctor's supervision. Marijuana is useful for many more disorders than most doctors realize. The federal government in the United States recognizes zero medical use for this medical substance even though cannabinoids offer front-line medicinal support for radiation exposure, cancer, diabetes, and a host of neurological conditions. It is also the best and safest all-purpose pain medication. Marijuana is effective in easing the inflammation of inflammatory bowel disease and is very beneficial in easing the spasticity of multiple sclerosis.

If you care about medicine, people's lives, and what they suffer through, you will be interested in studying marijuana and its use in the treatment of disease, not only physical syndromes but mental and emotional ones as well. Prof. Rafael Meshulam, an Israel Prize laureate for chemistry says that,

"Cannabis is a medicine in every respect." It is medically outrageous to exclude this substance from medical cabinets and pharmacies because only more dangerous medicines can be put in marijuana's place.

The compounds contained in cannabis possess therapeutic properties for a wide variety of human diseases and physical ailments. That is not all. Cannabis is a five-purpose plant: as a source of hempen fibres, for its oil, for its akenes or "seeds" consumed by man for food, for its narcotic properties, and therapeutically in medicine to treat a wide spectrum of ills.

Medicinal marijuana is now a mainstream method of treatment for many health issues. Cannabis is prescribed to glaucoma patients to relieve eye pressure and to sufferers of multiple sclerosis to stop or reduce muscle spasms. It is prescribed to cancer and AIDS patients to reduce nausea and stimulate appetite. Marijuana has also been used effectively to treat epilepsy, depression, and anxiety. However, that is only the beginning of the story.

The earliest record of the medicinal use of the plant is that of the Chinese emperor herbalist Shen Nung who, 5,000 years ago, recommended cannabis for malaria, beri-beri, constipation, rheumatic pains, absent-mindedness, and female disorders. Hoa-Glio, another ancient Chinese herbalist, recommended a mixture of hemp resin and wine as an analgesic during surgery.

The research indicates that cannabinoids hold the secret to helping heal many of the chronic diseases we are facing. From cancer to diabetes, and from autism to Alzheimer's, medical marijuana helps—sometimes dramatically so. Cannabinoid medicine holds a great power to alleviate human suffering. There are no words to describe how important this substance is for our race in terms of sanity, compassion, and highly rational medicine. I have said— and will continue to say in this book—the same about magnesium chloride, but for now this very interesting and powerful weed is on stage.

> *Signaling by the cannabinoid system represents a mechanism by which neurons can communicate backwards across synapses to modulate their inputs.*
>
> —DR. ROGER A. NICOLL, UCSF PROFESSOR OF CELLULAR
> AND MOLECULAR PHARMACOLOGY

A cannabinoid is the signaling molecule within a unique system of communication that is activated intermittently between two of the brain's most ubiquitous nerve cells—neurons containing the inhibitory neurotransmitter GABA and neurons containing the excitatory neurotransmitter glutamate. The modulation of inhibitory and excitatory signals leads to the regulation of excitation and inhibition within clusters of neurons that is the basis for all action and thought.

Present evidence suggests that the endocannabinoids and their receptors constitute a widespread modulatory system that fine-tunes bodily responses to a number of stimuli.

This mystery unraveled in 1964 when tetrahydrocannabinol, or THC, the main psychoactive chemical in cannabis, was isolated and synthesized by Raphael Mechoulam and colleagues in Israel. Subsequently in 1988, Allyn Howlett and colleagues discovered the cannabinoid receptor in the brain.

Dr. Melamede, Associate Professor and Biology Chairman, Biology Department, University of Colorado, explains that the endocannabinoid system functions as a "global homeostatic regulator," balancing organ systems. He theorizes that, "Free radicals are the friction of life. Endocannabinoids are the oil of life." Variously described as "super-modulator," "the normalizer" and "global homeostatic regulator," the endocannabinoid system is responsible for maintaining homeostasis—crucial balancing acts that the brain constantly performs in hormonal and endocrine systems, cellular chemistry, and organ systems all over the body.

Jeremiah Vandermeer takes us inside those sticky resinous growths known as trichomes, which are home to the active ingredients in cannabis. He says, "In nature, only the strong survive, and it is hypothesized by biologists that trichomes evolved as a defense mechanism of the cannabis plant against a range of potential enemies. Trichomes, from the Greek meaning 'growth of hair,' act as an evolutionary shield, protecting the plant and its seeds from the dangers of its environment, allowing it to reproduce. These adhesive sprouts form a protective layer against offensive insects, preventing them from reaching the surface of the plant. The chemicals in the trichomes make cannabis less palatable to hungry animals and can inhibit the growth of some types of fungus. The resin also helps to insulate the plant from high wind and low humidity, and acts as a natural 'sunscreen' in protecting against UV-B light rays."

Dr. Gregory T. Carter, Clinical Associate Professor of Rehabilitation Medicine, University of Washington School of Medicine, says, "Marijuana is a complex substance containing over 60 different forms of cannabinoids, the active ingredients. Cannabinoids are now known to have the capacity for neuromodulation via direct, receptor-based mechanisms at numerous levels within the nervous system. These have therapeutic properties that may be applicable to the treatment of neurological disorders, including anti-oxidative, neuroprotective, analgesic and anti-inflammatory actions, and immunomodulation, modulation of glial cells and tumor growth regulation. Intracellular changes and altered signaling of the neurons seems to be the principle effects of the cannabinoids in marijuana."

EMERGING CLINICAL APPLICATIONS FOR CANNABIS AND CANNABINOIDS

Medical marijuana, right now, is commonly used to alleviate nausea and chronic pain, but research indicates that cannabis has many other benefits. Marijuana is useful for many more disorders than most doctors realize. Cannabinoids offer front-line medicinal support for:

■ Alcohol abuse

■ Depression

■ Cancer

  • Stops breast cancer from spreading

  • Reduces tumors and kills brain cancer cells

  • Reduces tumors and slows growth of lung cancer cells

  • Leukemia

■ Diabetes

■ Neurological conditions

  • Bipolar disorder

  • Can help prevent the formation of Alzheimer's plaques in the brain

  • Epilepsy

  • Improves ability to concentrate in some cases of ADD

  • Parkinson's

  • Prevents loss of consciousness

■ Radiation exposure

It is also the best and safest all-purpose pain medication. Marijuana is effective in easing the inflammation of inflammatory bowel disease and is very beneficial in easing the spasticity of multiple sclerosis.

EFFECTIVE TREATMENTS

Dr. William Dale, section chief of geriatrics and palliative medicine at the University of Chicago Medical Center, said marijuana *raises users' heart rates and lowers their blood pressure.* Natural Allopathic Medicine mixes magnesium chloride in a protocol with cannabinoids to compete for the supreme medical choice of doctors who are struggling to keep their patients' blood pressure and stress levels down while simultaneously strengthening the heart with the extra help of iodine.

Magnesium chloride is a potent mineral medicine; it is safe and incredibly fast-acting, as is marijuana. When magnesium is combined with cannabinoid medicine we dramatically increase the medical horsepower we are applying and can expect superior results. For many conditions, using both together will yield results much greater than when using either alone. Magnesium is the lamp of life and without it we are toast! Cannabinoids tap into communication on cellular and intracellular levels like nothing else does, orchestrating changes in people not only on physical levels but also on emotional, mental, and spiritual plains of existence.

Medical Marijuana

Studies indicate that because of its broadband effect, cannabis can be used in almost all clinical and subclinical situations including lessening the suffering from a common cold. It can be used in the treatments of a number of diseases/disorders as well. (*See* Part 2)

Magnesium

Magnesium, especially when applied transdermally, is the medical miracle we have been waiting for and, when used to support the use of medical marijuana, takes us to a new level of safe and effective medical practice. Cannabinoids have been around forever and so has magnesium in the sea, but it is only recently that magnesium has been discovered for the beautiful medicine it is. The two together should be stocked in medicine cabinets providing the safest, most effective medicine team we can recommend for patients.

Magnesium and bicarbonate are used in emergency rooms and intensive care wards where they routinely save lives in a heartbeat when injected or used in IV drips. Marijuana is a medically useful substance that also can save lives as well as alleviate much suffering and pain.

CONCLUSION

Since the marijuana plant is composed of chemicals that help treat a range of disorders or their symptoms, one may argue that it should be legal for medical purposes. Modern research has shown that cannabis, along with magnesium, is a valuable aid in a wide range of treatments. As a result, a growing number of states have legalized marijuana for its medical use.

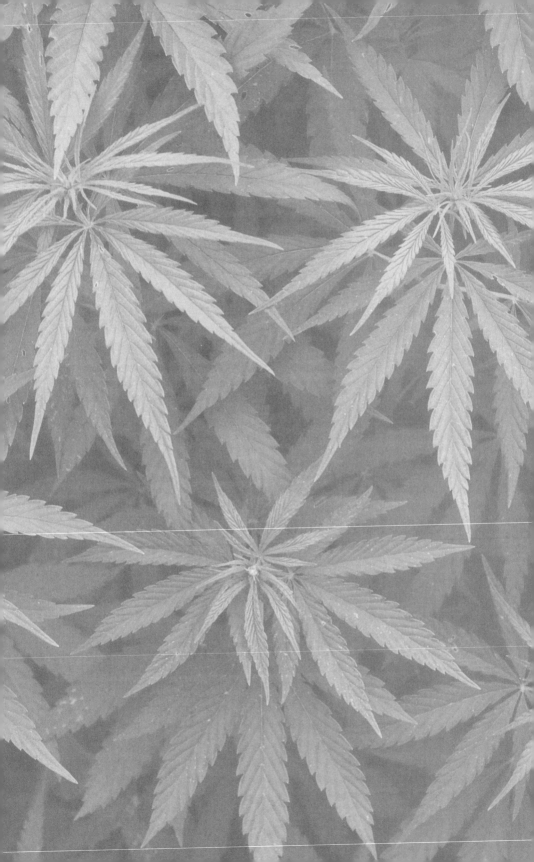

3.

Safe for Men, Women, and Children

In medicine we have the overriding concern of finding the very safest and most effective medicines and treatments. It is a sad world that the institution of medicine and pharmaceutical interests would replace marijuana with drugs so dangerous that they can make people violent and kill. The U.S. Food and Drug Administration (FDA) has not approved the use of natural cannabis as a treatment for any medical condition, but it *has* approved many drugs that kill over 100,000 people each and every year even when properly prescribed. Marijuana holds the heavyweight title for drug safety being that it's famous for *not* being the cause of death of *anyone*.

A Canadian judge ruled that Prozac was the cause that led a teenage high school student—with no prior history of violence—to inexplicably murder his friend with a single stab wound to the chest. The judge based his determination largely on the compelling expert testimony by US psychiatrist, Peter Breggin, MD who submitted scientific evidence showing the risk of drug-induced violence posed by antidepressants such as Prozac.

According to court documents, "The boy had been taking Prozac for three months, during which time his behavior deteriorated. He became impulsive and unpredictable, and suicidal. He also began to talk at times as if fantasizing about violence. He seemed to become a different person to his distraught parents." The judge was also persuaded by the fact that when Prozac was withdrawn from the boy, his behavior returned to normal.

Dr. Breggin testified that his primary care physician and his parents alerted the prescribing psychiatric clinic to the boy's deteriorating condition, but the clinic continued the Prozac and then doubled it. This is the first criminal case in North America where a judge has specifically found that an antidepressant was the cause of a murder.

Dr. Breggin noted that: "This is a landmark legal confirmation of the scientific fact that the newer antidepressants like Prozac, including the SSRI and SNRI antidepressants, can cause violence and even murder."

In another case:

In June 2001, a jury ordered GlaxoSmithKline, the maker of Paxil, to pay $6.5 million to the relatives of Donald Schell, who, two days after starting on the drug, murdered his wife, his daughter and his grand-daughter before killing himself. Christopher Pittman, who at 12 years of age killed both his grandparents, is said to have done so for a reason beyond the boy's control—a reaction to the antidepressant Zoloft, a drug he had started taking for depression not long before the slaying.

> *Christopher committed the murders*
> *while in a psychotic state induced by Zoloft.*
> —DR. LANETTE ATKINS, FORENSIC PSYCHIATRIST

The official medical world as represented by the United States government—and most others for that matter—prefer dangerous carcinogenic substances over safe, effective, and natural substances like marijuana. Some people might doubt such a safety claim saying, "somewhere someone who was using marijuana too heavily must have perished" and they are probably right. We could also say that probably someone somewhere in the world dies from choking on water every day, yet the safety of drinking water is never challenged. Although marijuana can be addictive, addiction rates are often lower than those to opioid drugs, and discontinuing the use of marijuana is not associated with the severe withdrawal symptoms experience with the withdrawal of opioids.

HOW SAFE IS MEDICAL MARIJUANA?

"Marijuana has remarkably low toxicity and lethal doses in humans have not been described. This is in stark contrast to a number of commonly prescribed medications used for similar purposes, including opiates, anti-emetics, anti-depressants, and muscle relaxants, not to mention legal substances used recreationally, including tobacco and alcohol," writes Dr. Gregory T. Carter, Clinical Associate Professor of Rehabilitation Medicine, University of Washington School of Medicine. Notice Dr. Carter said low toxicity not no toxicity.

"It seems to me if one is going to need to use drugs, one ought to consider a relatively safe drug, like marijuana," said Bernard Rimland, PhD of the Autism Research Institute. Marijuana, the forbidden medicine, seems to be useful for some people with adult attention deficit disorder, impulse disorders, and bipolar disorder. Many families have found marijuana to be nothing short of miraculous. Some of the symptoms marijuana has ameliorated include anxiety—even severe anxiety—aggression, panic disorder, generalized rage, tantrums, and self-injurious behavior. Patients report medical marijuana as more therapeutic and better tolerated than other medications.

Cannabinoids are usually well tolerated, and do not produce the generalized toxic effects of conventional pharmaceuticals but that does not mean we do not have to be careful with its long-term use. At Columbia University's National Center on Addiction and Substance Abuse, where a great deal of National Institute for Drug Abuse (NIDA) funded research takes place, researchers have found that abrupt marijuana withdrawal leads to symptoms similar to depression and nicotine withdrawal. Meaning that no matter how helpful marijuana is as a medicine it is not without its own toxicity and addictive properties. Marijuana is a complex substance affecting each person differently.

> I am 55 and I have been smoking pot off and on for the last 30 years... I had no idea of the withdrawal I would experience. Two days in, I thought for sure I had some dreaded disease. One minute I would be freezing, the next sweating. The loss of appetite doesn't bother me because pot always helped me keep on an extra 5 to 10 lbs from the munchies and sweet tooth. Not sure how long it will take, but I do look forward to the day when this has all passed.

Long-term use or overuse of marijuana has been linked to adrenal fatigue, sexual dysfunctions, and it has effects on the brain cells that cause short-term memory loss. Marijuana itself usually does not cause liver damage, but most marijuana contains various impurities and other plant material that can be damaging to the liver. One way to tell if it is bothering your liver is if you start feeling dizzy and having trouble walking when taking marijuana. Another way you can tell is if the liver itself and the area above it on the rib cage becomes sensitive to the touch. That said a low risk profile is evident from the literature available. Serious complications are very rare and are not usually reported during the use of cannabinoids for medical indications.

Years ago, the American College of Physicians (ACP) issued a policy statement endorsing medical marijuana use. The group has urged the government in the past to reverse its ban on medical treatments using marijuana. "ACP encourages the use of non-smoked forms of THC that have proven therapeutic value," the new policy statement said. The Philadelphia-based organization, the second largest doctors group in the United States, cited studies into marijuana's medical applications, such as treating severe weight loss associated with illnesses such as AIDS and treating nausea and vomiting associated with chemotherapy for cancer patients.

HOW SAFE IS MEDICAL MARIJUANA FOR CHILDREN?

The idea of using medical marijuana as treatment for a child still gives pause to many adults who associate the drug with recreational use that breaks the law. One mother commenting on using marijuana for her autistic child said, "I know it's not the end all answer, but it's been the best answer for the longest time for us in regards to *all* the other medications. I cannot tell you how many months we would go on a medication wondering if it was doing anything, anything at all. Here we can see the difference in 30 to 60 minutes guaranteed."

Rick Simpson, the author of *Phoenix Tears—The Rick Simpson Story,* says, "I know of nothing better than hemp oil to prevent diseases. I consider hemp to be perfectly safe in the treatment of children. I have often stated that if children were given tiny doses of hemp oil, diseases like diabetes, MS, cancer, and many others could be prevented from ever occurring. If minute doses of oil are given to children, THC and its associated cannabinoids will build up in their systems and prevent disease. I am not talking about getting children high; this is about providing children with a harmless, non-addictive medicine to prevent disease. Just like it must have been in history—do you think they did not give children the medication that they knew worked best? As for doses, children are no different than adults; they all have different tolerances for this medication. To prevent diseases in children, only minuscule doses would be required, so the chance of getting a child high would be very remote."

SIDE EFFECTS, WARNINGS, AND CONTRAINDICATIONS

Marijuana, depending on the growing, storage, and handling conditions, can contain fungal contaminants that can be problematic in already immune-compromised people. Most people who are healthy have immune systems that can deal with these fungi, but if your health is compromised, the ingestion of the fungi often found in marijuana leaves and buds can become a problem and even develop into an infection that can be dangerous.

Damp marijuana is the perfect breeding ground for aspergilla and many thousands of other molds (and bacteria). Aspergillosis is the most common fungal infection in marijuana smokers caused by aspergilla fumigates.

Dr. Gabriel Cousens writes, "While marijuana may have many palliative qualities, the psychoactive species have some serious downsides. As he points out, "Marijuana's side effects increase over time" and are cumulative. He has clinically observed that "marijuana's effects can have a drying and toxic quality. They tend to take a general progression from the lungs to the digestion and immune systems, then to the blood, heart and circulatory system, then on to the liver and nervous systems and finally to the sexual, endocrine systems and brain over time."

Marijuana, however, usually gives more than it takes from the body, mind, and emotions when used as a medicine. Marijuana has a large benefit curve that varies greatly depending not only on a person's presenting condition but also on their character and inner strength. Over time though, sometimes a great deal of time, this curve reverses, and it may begin to take more than it gives meaning side effects can creep up to disturb the body, mind, and spirit. What can we expect from a substance that greatly affects our brain wave patterns? If a person keeps taking marijuana over years, he may become dependent, addicted, and eventually may lose the ability to cope with its toxicity. This dependency varies widely from one person to another and for some never becomes a threat to their health or quality of life.

Some people notice an increasing sense of restlessness when they get high. This is direct feedback from their bodies telling them that something's wrong. Most people just go ahead ignoring the body's feedback signals. This in and of itself creates a biological stress inside a person, creating trauma. The body has to cope; we give it no choice when we ignore negative symptoms. A price is taken out of the central nervous system creating what John Mini M.S.C.M./L.Ac. calls *Marijuana Induced Stress Trauma*.

There are people who have had bad experiences with marijuana. Marijuana is not a pure and regulated substance—the strains are all different, the growing conditions, the drying and storage conditions are all different—and these things affect how that pot will affect a person. Immune suppressed people have to be careful what they smoke or where they get it or a drastic infection could override any benefit the pot may give them.

Diabetes

Appetite stimulation can be dangerous for diabetics, especially for those needing to lose weight. Currently research is attempting to find an effective CB1 (cannabinoid receptor antagonist) that will counter the effects of THC of increasing hunger in Type-2 diabetics. Decreases in blood sugars (hypoglycemia) can go unrecognized due to the psychoactive effects of the THC. Untreated low blood sugar leads to the loss of consciousness and seizures.

Yet a study published in the *American Journal of Medicine* in 2013 shows that "current marijuana use was associated with 16 percent lower fasting insulin levels . . . and 17 percent lower HOMA-IR (insulin resistance). We found significant associations between marijuana use and smaller waist circumferences."

Murray Mittleman, Associate Professor of Medicine at Harvard Medical School and the study's lead author, told *Time* magazine last year that "the most important finding is that current users of marijuana appeared to have better carbohydrate metabolism than nonusers. "Their fasting insulin levels were lower, and they appeared to be less resistant to the insulin produced by their body to maintain a normal blood-sugar level."

Cardiovascular System

Tachycardia and hypotension are frequently documented as adverse events in the cardiovascular system. A few cases of myocardial ischemia have been reported in young and previously healthy patients. Inhaling the smoke of cannabis cigarettes induces side effects on the respiratory system. Cannabinoids are contraindicated for patients with a history of cardiac ischemias.

Nervous System

Unstable people can become unglued after smoking marijuana, though the effects are normally temporary. Cannabinoids can exacerbate schizophrenic psychosis in persons predisposed to such. Cannabinoids impede cognitive and psychomotor performance, resulting in temporary impairment. Chronic use can lead to the development of tolerance.

Marijuana does not have to do physical damage to a person's nervous system to affect the way it functions. The more a person denies their feelings and what their body is telling them to do, the deeper the traumatic split goes into the nervous system.

Digestive System

A large part of marijuana's direct influence affects the stomach and pancreas. This is what gives people the munchies. Various digestive issues may enter into the picture along the way that can be equally difficult to treat if one continues abusing marijuana. The higher the THC content in smoked marijuana is, the greater is the effect of hunger (munchies)—this will exacerbate the problem of obesity and insulin resistance.

RISING POTENCY

The amount of THC in marijuana samples confiscated by police has been increasing steadily over the past few decades. In 2012, THC concentrations in marijuana averaged close to 15 percent, compared to around 4 percent in the 1980s. For a new user, this may mean exposure to higher concentrations of THC, with a greater chance of an adverse or unpredictable reaction. Increases in potency may account for the rise in emergency department visits involving marijuana use. For frequent users, it may mean a greater risk for addiction if they are exposing themselves to high doses on a regular basis. However, the full range of consequences associated with marijuana's higher potency is not well understood.

Cadmium concentrates in tobacco and marijuana leaves and accumulates in the body when smoked over a long term leading to hypertension, kidney degeneration or disease, heart disease, depressed immune systems, cancers of the lungs and prostate; it also affects bones. In healthy people excess cadmium can be excreted in the urine if adequate levels of zinc are maintained in the body—15 to 30 mg daily in a supplement, will offer some protection against cadmium problems.

IF YOU DECIDE TO STOP USING MARIJUANA

You may decide that the effects on your body are becoming more detrimental in your use of marijuana. When this happens, there are many treatment options available and programs spring up all over the place with pharmaceutical drugs and numerous supplements to help people get off marijuana. Many people will find it easier to enter these programs, but you can also safely withdraw at home.

John Mini, author of *Marijuana Syndromes*, tells us, "You can tell if a person is physically addicted to marijuana if he/she hasn't had marijuana for a while and he/she feels withdrawal symptoms. These symptoms can come in the forms of depression, irritability, anxiety, trouble sleeping, emotional neediness, or nausea."

Margaret Hanley, PhD from Columbia University makes these recommendations if you decide you want to stop using marijuana: "If one wants to detox on one's own, it is good to go into it prepared to experience withdrawal symptoms, such as disrupted sleep, decreased food intake, irritable mood, decreased sociability, and marijuana craving. Most symptoms peak around 3 to 4 days without smoking, but symptoms can last for over a week."

THC is stored in the fat tissues and can even remain there for over a month. To help to detoxify, an adequate exercise program that burns fat and increase in water intake will help to flush out the THC by-products from your body. Drink as much good quality water as possible. This kind of natural remedy can dispense these by-products from your system in less than a week, but it may take longer in long term heavy marijuana users.

Avoid any pharmaceutical medicines. Take a source of good natural whole food vitamins and minerals. Acupuncture will help, as well as daily or even multiple magnesium massages each day during the worst periods of withdrawal.

CONCLUSION

One of the benefits of treating disorders and diseases with medical marijuana is its safety record; there is no known case of a lethal overdose. It can also be less addictive than many other drugs prescribed today, such as muscle relaxants, hypnotics, and analgesics. However, cannabis is not a completely harmless substance; it can have various physiological effects and adverse effects as mentioned in this chapter.

4.

Medical Marijuana in Pediatric Medicine

Not many people or physicians realize how useful or even critical medical marijuana can be in pediatrics—or how it can save many children's lives. We are talking about serious medicine and the pharmaceutical companies know this and are making synthetic versions of THC, but synthetic copies cannot compete with the real thing in terms of safety and effectiveness.

Many physicians, even in California, refrain from approving use of cannabis by patients out of residual fear. Countless others refrain because they learned nothing about cannabis in medical school and cannot knowledgeably advise patients about dosage, side effects, or mechanism of action. This is of course not an acceptable situation, especially in pediatric care, because it is so useful and safe and potentially lifesaving in certain cases.

Recently, researcher Dr. Ester Fride of the Behavioral Sciences Department of Israel's College of Judea and Samaria, published a pair of scientific papers stating that the brain's cannabinoid receptors (receptors in the brain that respond pharmacologically to various compounds in cannabis as well as other endogenous compounds), and the naturally occurring messenger molecules that activate and bind to them (so-called endocannabinoids) "are present from the early stages of gestation" and may play "a number of vital roles" in human prenatal and postnatal development.

Writing in *Neuroendocrinology Letters* and the *European Journal of Pharmacology*, Fride suggests, "A role for the endocannabinoid system for the human infant is likely." She notes that in animals, the endogenous cannabinoid system fulfills several important developmental functions, including embryonal implantation (which requires a temporary and localized reduction in the production of the endocannabinoid anandamide), neural development, neuroprotection, the development of memory and oral-motor skills, and the initiation of suckling in newborns. A dysfunctional endocannabinoid system, Fride speculates, may be responsible for certain abnormalities in infants, particularly "failure-to-thrive" syndrome, a condition in which newborns fail to properly grow and gain weight. (In animal studies, mice fail to gain weight and die within the first week of life when their cannabinoid receptors are blocked.)

Dr. Fride strongly recommends the use of cannabinoids in pediatric medicine. She notes that "excellent clinical results" have been reported in pediatric oncology and in case studies of children with severe neurological diseases or brain trauma, and suggests that cannabis-derived medicines could also play a role in the treatment of other childhood syndromes, including the pain and gastrointestinal inflammation associated with cystic fibrosis. Because the development of the cannabinoid receptor system appears to occur gradually over the course of childhood, "children may be less prone to the psychoactive side effects of THC or endocannabinoids than adults,"

Fride writes. "Therefore, it is suggested that children may respond positively to the medicinal applications of cannabinoids without [psychoactive] effects." She concludes, "The medical implications of these novel developments are far reaching and suggest a promising future for cannabinoids in pediatric medicine" for conditions including cachexia (severe weight loss), cystic fibrosis, failure-to-thrive, anorexia, inflammation, and chronic pain.

"It's clear that the cannabinoid system is essential for complete human development, and that cannabis medicines have a great potential to help sick children," says University of Southern California Professor Mitch Earlywine, author of the book, *Understanding Marijuana: A New Look at the Scientific Evidence*. "Given the well-established safety of the medication, clinical trials for other disorders, particularly cystic fibrosis and 'failure-to-thrive,' seem a humane and essential next step."

ADHD

"It's safer than aspirin," Dr. Talleyrand said. He and other marijuana advocates maintain that it is also safer than methylphenidate (Ritalin), the stimulant prescription drug most often used to treat ADHD (Attention Deficit Hyperactivity Disorder). That drug has documented potential side effects, including insomnia, depression, facial tics, and stunted growth. Marijuana is "a godsend" for some people with ADHD, said Dr. Edward M. Hallowell, a psychiatrist who has written several books on the disorder.

Several Bay Area doctors who recommend medical marijuana for their patients said in recent interviews that their client base had expanded to include teenagers with psychiatric conditions, including ADHD. Dr. Jean Talleyrand, who founded MediCann, a network in Oakland of 20 clinics who authorize patients to use the drug, said his staff members had treated as many as 50 patients ages 14 to 18 with ADHD.

In Berkeley, Dr. Frank Lucido authorized marijuana for a 16-year-old boy with ADHD who had tried Ritalin unsuccessfully and was racking up a record of minor arrests. Within a year of the new treatment, he said, the boy was getting better grades and was even elected president of his special-education class. "He was telling his mother: 'My brain works. I can think'," Dr. Lucido said.

Pharmaceutical companies are all in favor of drugging preschoolers with Ritalin even though about 40 percent of children developed side effects and roughly 11 percent dropped out because of problems including irritability, weight loss, insomnia, and slowed growth. "Preschoolers on methylphenidate, or generic Ritalin, grew about half an inch less and gained about two pounds less than expected during the 70-week study. This is a catastrophe. It just opens up the way for drugging the younger kids," said Dr. Peter Breggin, a New York psychiatrist and longtime critic of psychiatric drug use in children. Breggin said the research is part of a marketing push by the drug industry to expand drug use to the youngest children.

AUTISM

Knocking on death's door, 10-year-old Joey P. was slowly dying. The potpourri of prescription medications he'd consumed since the age of five had damaged his body beyond repair—the side effects were literally killing him. Joey was diagnosed with autism at 18 months old. At one point, he was taking six different medications—up to three times a day. As a result of the side effects, Joey became malnourished and was diagnosed with anorexia. Every day, his condition got worse. His eyes were sunken in and you could easily see all the bones in his chest. He was refusing to eat.

At the end of his allopathic treatments his medical prognosis was high probability of death within six months. Today, Joey is thriving and his mother has been on *The Good Morning Show* to share that the compassionate use of medical marijuana saved her son's life.

"Although medical marijuana is not known to be a cure for autism, it has been proven to facilitate 'life' for my son and has ushered him into his most progressive developmental period ever.

Today at age 11, Joey is flourishing with new communicative expressions, he's gained over 40 pounds, and he's happier, healthier, better behaved, and is more productively active than ever before. Before we began to give him treatments of oral marijuana he was a danger to himself and others. He had suffered from anxiety, OCD (obsessive-compulsive disorder), and aggression since an early age. At the age 5, Joey was prescribed the first of many ineffective, harmful medications. The medications he was prescribed at that time worked for about a year, but Joey refused to eat and that was the beginning of their story. As a result of the serious side effects, Joey became malnourished and was diagnosed with anorexia. It was the famous marijuana brownies that saved my son's life, and it was the doctors and their pharmaceutical medicines that almost killed him." (*See* Part 2 page 98)

CANCER

Dr. Linda Granowetter was quoted as saying, "We know from research that 30 to 60 percent of parents are giving their children alternative meds like vitamins, shark cartilage, and herbs from Chinatown. That's why we spend a lot of time asking parents what else they are giving kids and trying to be non-judgmental and work with them and guide them." She said most pediatric oncologists are "open-minded" about alternative treatments (*see* Part 2 page 100).

Marijuana was the best medicine for 3-year-old Cash Hyde of Missoula, Montana. The boy's parent's defied doctor's orders—and Montana law—to get their hands on the medicinal treatment their son needed after he was diagnosed with recurring brain tumors at 22 months old. "I've had law enforcement threatening to kick my door down, but I would have done anything to keep Cashy alive," Mike Hyde, the boy's father said to ABCNews.com.

Please note in the story on *ABC News* that Mike Hyde made his own hemp oil, *see* page 31.

Rick Simpson, who continues to be a rock of integrity about the use of hemp oil for the cure of cancer, warns people to make it themselves because the quality of purchased oil is highly questionable. Simpson said:

> That's the reason I tell the public it's best to produce your own oil at this time, until we have some standards in place. If you produce the oil yourself, at least then you know you have the real thing and to a dying patient, the proper oil can mean the difference between life and death.
>
> The public must realize that all hemp is not created equal; the medicinal qualities from strain to strain can vary a great deal so the proper strains must be used. Also low-grade strains and clippings may produce a decent treatment for some skin conditions. But if you are trying to treat someone with a serious condition like cancer, low-grade oils just don't cut it; only the best will do.
>
> These are trying times for us all, but soon things will settle down and the public will have their medicine. It's just a matter of time now, for there is no way for the system to stop the truth from spreading. Properly produced hemp oil is the greatest medicine on this earth, and soon hemp will again take its rightful place in mainstream medicinal use.

Marijuana Saves Baby from Cancer

A 2011 article from ABC News reported the story of a two-year-old boy with a stage 4 brain tumor who was successfully treated with marijuana. The boy, Cash Hyde, had cancer so severe that he had experienced septic shock, a stroke, pulmonary hemorrhaging, and blindness due to the tumor impeding his optic nerve. Working with his doctors, seven different chemotherapy drugs were used, to little avail.

For two months, the little boy was given the maximum doses of chemotherapy. He lost his appetite, threw up several times a day, and had even stopped eating for forty days. That was when his father, Mike Hyde, decided to intervene. "He was suffering terribly, and the doctors said it was the best they could do for him," said Hyde, who ordered that the chemotherapy drugs be stopped.

The Hydes are from Missoula, Montana, a state in which medical marijuana is legal. Mike obtained a marijuana card for Cash and produced his own cannabis oil. He boiled the marijuana with olive oil and slipped 3 mm doses into his son's feeding tube twice a day. Cash miraculously recovered at Primary Children's Hospital in Salt Lake City, Utah (a state in which marijuana is not legal), but his father's unauthorized treatment stirred debate about a parent's role in medical treatment—a debate that continues to this day.

Nevertheless, Mike did not regret his decision to go behind doctors' backs and against Utah law in treating his son: ". . . it was a godsend . . . In two weeks, he was weaned of all the nausea drugs, and he was eating again and sitting up and laughing." Hyde added that doctors called Cash's recovery "a miracle."

Raw Michelle cited a case where medical marijuana is the right choice for medical treatment:

At two years old, Amber was diagnosed with terminal brain tumors. Her mother was told that with treatment, Amber had a 10 percent chance of survival. After surgery, radiation, and chemotherapy, the tumors were still spreading. Her parents were advised to take their child home, make her comfortable, and prepare for the inevitable. A month later, her parents reported a startling change. The tumors had decreased in size and number. The family had been **juicing cannabis leaves and feeding their baby a few ounces of the juice each day.**

CONCLUSION

The stigma associated with "marijuana" presents powerful discouragement to doctors. Although the medical community, such as the American Academy of Pediatrics (AAP), opposes the legalization of medical marijuana for children, they recently have advocated for research using medical marijuana for treating symptoms that are not presently relieved by the recommended drugs.

5.

Therapeutic Cannabis Dosages

There are no exact doses or existing fixed dosing schedules for fresh marijuana, smoked/vaporized marijuana, or cannabis oil. The required dosage to attain therapeutic effects and to stay clear from adverse effects is difficult to estimate and is affected by many factors. Nonetheless, higher doses of THC and CBD are related to an increased chance of encountering adverse or harmful effects. The quantity remains highly personalized and relies to a great degree on titration (the strength, measure); trying to find the right dose where potential positive therapeutic effects are maximized and adverse or harmful effects are minimized. The most sensible approach choosing a dose when no evidence-based guideline exists is to begin with a low dose and proceed slowly.

Donald Abrams, MD, Professor of Clinical Medicine at the University of California, San Francisco, et al., in their research paper "Medical Cannabis: Rational Guidelines for Dosing," published January 2004 on CannabisMD.org, wrote:

> An experienced cannabis smoker can titrate and regulate dose to obtain the desired acute effects and to minimize undesired effects. Each puff delivers a discrete dose of cannabinoids to the body. Puff and inhalation volume changes with phase of smoking, tending to be highest at the beginning and lowest at the end of smoking a cigarette...Oral ingestion of THC or cannabis has quite different pharmacokinetics than inhalation. The onset of action is delayed and titration of dosing is more difficult.

Chris Conrad in an essay entitled "Cannabis Yields and Dosages" agrees, stating:

> The means of ingestion also affects patient dosage. Smoked cannabis provides rapid and efficient delivery. Most patients consume it this way,

but some wish to avoid the smoke. "Vaporizing" it (heat without combustion) may require twice as much. NIDA [National Institute on Drug Abuse] estimates that eating requires three to five times the smoked dosage.

This means that a patient who smokes a pound per year needs about four pounds for the same effect if they eat it, although often they prefer a combination of the two. When eaten, cannabis' effects are spread out over a longer period of time. This may be particularly good for sleep or situations where smoking is impractical or impossible, but due to its delayed onset and varied metabolic activity, eaten is hard to titrate. Consumable goods spoil over time, there is a learning curve to prepare recipes, and not every attempt produces usable medicine. Making kef, hash, tinctures, oil, extracts, topical salves, and liniment all require ample amounts of cannabis. Patients need an accurate scale to measure, track, and titrate their own personal dosage and supply of cannabis.

Thus, a patient-determined, self-titrated dosing model is recommended. This self-titration model is acceptable given the heretofore-discussed variables as well as the low toxicity of cannabis. This construct is not unique to cannabis. Many other drugs have relatively low toxicity and high dosing ceilings (gabapentin being one notable example) and are titrated to effect.

Dosing of medical cannabis has been determined through elaborate scientific analysis of the most prominent cannabinoid, THC.

In a 1999 lecture at the Lindesmith Center in San Francisco, Dr. Abrams noted:

When taken by mouth, delta-9 THC has a very low 6 to 20 percent absorption, and it's very variable from one person to another. Peak plasma concentrations of delta-9 THC, when taken by mouth, occur within one to six hours and may remain elevated for several hours with a half-life of 20 to 30 hours. So it sticks around for a long time. It takes a long time to reach a peak concentration. Similarly, when taken by mouth, delta-9 THC is broken down into the liver to a by-product of 11 hydroxyl THC, it's called, which in and of itself, this metabolite, has potent psychoactive effects. You get less of it when you smoke it... The 11 hydroxyl, which in and of itself is a potent metabolite, and when smoked you produce less of the 11 hydroxyl. Smoking THC, the THC is rapidly absorbed into the blood stream and redistributed with a considerable amount of it destroyed by combustion. Peak plasma levels are achieved at the very end of smoking and decline rapidly over 30 minutes, as if it were given intravenously, for example, whereas, if taken by mouth, it's slow and doesn't reach very high peaks and takes a long time to disappear. The amount of THC one is exposed to might be the same, but certainly the effects are different.

A U.S. Office of National Drug Control Policy (ONDCP) senior speechwriter, Kevin A. Sabet, told ProCon.org in a January 22, 2004 email: "Smoked marijuana has no reliable dosage . . ." Jay Cavanaugh, PhD, National Director of the American Alliance for Medical Cannabis, wrote to ProCon.org on May 21, 2002 and said:

> When patients smoke or vaporize cannabis they can titrate their dose by inhalation. The medicinal constituents are absorbed in the lungs and proceed directly to the brain and general circulation avoiding a first pass through the liver. Patients can ascertain the effectiveness of the medicine within just a minute or two. By waiting between inhalations, patients can achieve the maximum effect with the least possible side effects.
>
> It is vitally important for naive patients (ones who haven't used cannabis socially or recreationally) to be trained by skilled caregivers into how to obtain the best relief with medication that may vary in potency from crop to crop or even in the same cannabis depending upon its age and moisture content. "Cured" cannabis, for instance, contains higher levels of THC and lower levels of CBD than fresh.

Dr. Mary Lynch, a pain researcher and head of the Canadian Consortium for the Investigation of Cannabinoids in Human Therapeutics, says there is very little research to guide practice so it's best to start with the lowest dose possible, particularly for the "naïve" (first-time) user. Using the protocols she and colleagues are developing for their research on the medicinal use of smoked marijuana, she recommends that naïve users begin with one puff (or toke), usually before bed, to help with symptoms, such as pain or spasticity and improve sleep quality. To get the most out of a dose while limiting the amount of smoke exposure, she tells patients to inhale on the pipe or joint and hold it in their lungs as long as possible.

Experienced users often know what dose is most effective, though Lynch recommends that a dose of 2 to 4 puffs per dose, 3 times per day is reasonable and, depending on response, the dose can be titrated accordingly. (Health Canada has suggested a daily maximum dose of 5 grams.) Much more information on dosing of cannabis can be found at the website listed in the Resource on Page 179.

Excerpted from that site:

Along with basic differences in individual metabolisms, various degrees of disease development, and even discounting the tolerance factor, there are distinct pharmacological differences among the many strains of cannabis in use today. THC is one of the active substances found in the resin of marijuana flowers. A handful of compounds called "cannabinoids" work together in a synergy of effects. Cannabis is one of the most diverse plant species cultivated, and there are subtle differences in the medicinal properties in use today. Such differences in medical effectiveness of various types of marijuana certainly alter the amounts required. It is also clear that potency is partially determined by cultivation techniques, which is another important variable in the range of quantities needed for various medical uses.

California NORML (National Association for Reform of Marijuana Laws) published the only reputable assay of medical marijuana in 1999. Those test results show a wide disparity in potency. "The study, consisting of three rounds of testing by two different DEA-licensed laboratories, measured the concentrations of THC, the primary active ingredient of marijuana, and its two commonest chemical relatives, known as cannabinoids, CBD and CBN. In all, 49 samples of medicinal cannabis were analyzed for potency by standard gas chromatograph mass spectrometry. "The sample showing the lowest THC (less than or equal to 3.9 percent) was the government's own marijuana, grown for the National Institute on Drug Abuse (NIDA) to supply researchers and eight legal medical marijuana patients. Nearly all other samples tested over 8 percent, with averages in the range of 12.8 percent to 15.4 percent, and many samples above 20 percent. One sample of hashish (concentrated resin) tested above 44 percent."

Some legal authorities might like to impose an exact and standardized dose limit that would apply universally in every case. Yet medical facts indicate that such a precise understanding may never be attained. Some patients use vastly greater amounts than others, and patients often develop patterns of use that may change with time due to numerous individual factors. Cannabis is non-toxic and there is no serious health risks associated with overdose, so the determination of dose limitations is primarily a concern of law enforcement. However, there has been inadequate scientific study of cannabis to firmly establish exact quantity limits for effective medical use at this time.

Some marijuana sold on the streets may also contain additives such as animal tranquilizers, often the only active ingredient in the product sold. On many forums it is reported that weed is mixed with such things as resins, sugar, PCP, LSD, cocaine, and other substances. Choose a reliable source! Most medical marijuana dispensaries do not sell cannabis mixed with other drugs or substances.

> *"Its margin of safety is immense and underscores the lack of any meaningful danger in using not only daily doses in the 3.5 to 9-gram range but also considerably higher doses."*
> —DAVID BEARMAN, M.D., PHYSICIAN, RESEARCHER,
> COURT-QUALIFIED CANNABIS EXPERT

Chronic pain patients tend to use larger amounts, while acute and terminal patients may use less. Conditions like glaucoma or MS may require continuous use to prevent attacks. Health conditions may periodically or cyclically improve or get worse, causing usage to fall or rise. Some require daily and multiple-daily dosages. **It is advisable to start with a low dose to avoid negative responses, especially when cannabis is eaten, and find your effective dose.**

Heavy smokers may experience respiratory irritation that can be minimized through vaporizing instead. Vaporizing generally requires a larger amount of marijuana to achieve medical benefit.

FOR ALZHEIMER'S AND OTHER NEUROLOGICAL DISEASES

> *The daily administration of 2.5 mg of synthetic THC over a two-week period reduced nocturnal motor activity and agitation in AD patients in an open-label pilot study.*
> —BERLIN GERMANY'S CHARITE UNIVERSITY,
> DEPARTMENT OF PSYCHIATRY AND PSYCHOTHERAPY

According to Gary Wenk, PhD, author of a December 2008 study and Professor of Psychology and Neuroscience at Ohio State University, "A puff is enough." He goes on to say that although this dose would probably have some sort of psychoactive effect, strictly medical use is not ruled out. The drug could be taken before bedtime, Wenk says, and with long-term use, tolerance to these psychoactive effects can develop, so impairment would be minimal with a steady dose and when taken this way.

Don Abrams, M.D., chief of hematology/oncology at San Francisco General Hospital, who has studied medical marijuana use in people with HIV for more than a decade stated: "Cannabis is anti-inflammatory and it is also an antioxidant, and those are two things that we seek in treating neurodegenerative disorders. It's there, it's in nature, if the research does find that it has these benefits, why not take advantage of it?"

> *Oral administration of up to 10 mg of synthetic THC*
> *reduced agitation and stimulated weight gain in late-stage*
> *Alzheimer's patients in an open-label clinical trial.*
> —INTERNATIONAL PSYCHOGERIATRIC ASSOCIATION

In 1974, the average THC content of illicit marijuana was less than one percent. Today most commercial grade marijuana from Mexico/Columbia and domestic outdoor cultivated marijuana has an average THC content of about 4 to 6 percent. Superior strains are being produced but are destined for medical use. Studies show stronger cannabis has a lower tar-to-weight ratio than weaker cannabis. An increase in cannabis potency may be viewed as a threat by the U.S. government, but it is a boon for medical users.

Chris Conrad, internationally known cannabis consultant who has testified as an expert witness in dozens of California marijuana cases, said, "You want to get the THC compounds while minimizing the amount of smoke and exposure to potentially carcinogenic matter. It is an odd thing to argue that medicines should be weaker."

> *The House of Lords in England has written about marijuana*
> *and has stated that not a single death can be attributed to its*
> *use anywhere on the planet. That would make marijuana*
> *the absolute safest medicine available today.*

SATIVA OR INDICA STRAINS

The effects of marijuana can vary greatly depending on which sub-species, or strain, you medicate with. The plant species Cannabis sativa L. has two main sub-species used for medicinal purposes: Cannabis indica and Cannnabis sativa.

Indica Strain

Indica strains are sedatives/relaxants and are effective for treating the symptoms of medical conditions such as:

- Anxiety
- Chronic Pain
- Insomnia
- Muscle Spasms
- Tremors

Indicas have a higher level of cannabinoids than sativas, which results in a sedated body-type stone. Because indica strains may cause feelings of sleepiness and heaviness, many patients prefer to medicate with this type of cannabis at night.

Effects of Indica (lower THC, higher CBN/CBD)

Indica's effects are generally more physical than cerebral (however, the relief of physical symptoms can have a positive psychological effect).

- Best for later in the day and bedtime
- Perhaps better for anxiety than depression
- Sedation, pain relief, and relaxation

Benefits of Indica (lower THC, higher CBN/CBD)

- Aids sleep
- Bronchio-dilator and expectorant
- Muscle relaxant
- Reduces anxiety and stress
- Relieves headaches and migraines
- Reduces intra-occular pressure
- Reduces inflammation
- Reduces inflammation
- Reduces pain
- Relieves spasms and reduces seizures
- Stimulates appetite

Sativa Strain

Sativa strains are more of a stimulant, and are effective in appetite stimulation, relieving depression, migraines, chronic pain, and nausea. Sativas have a higher level of THC than indicas, which results in a psychoactive and energetic mind-high. Because sativa strains may cause feelings of alertness and optimism, many patients prefer to medicate with this type of cannabis during the day.

Effects of Sativa (high THC, low CBN/CBD)

- Best for use in daytime
- Energizing and thought provoking
- Increases focus and creativity
- More stimulating and uplifting
- Supports immune system

Benefits of Sativa (high THC, low CBN/CBD)

- Acts as an expectorant
- Energizes and stimulates

- Fights drepression
- Positive, uplifting, cerebral effect
- Promotes creativity

- Relaxes muscles and relieves pain
- Relieves headaches and migraines
- Stimulates the appetite

Hybrids

Most cannabis seeds and medicine available today are from hybrids. Hybrids and cross-breeds of indica and sativa strains produce varieties that carry some characteristics of each parent. For example, adding sativa to indica strains adds mental clarity and decreases sedation effects. And adding indica to sativa strains can decrease or even eliminate the sativa tendency to stimulate anxiety.

Hybrids are often referred to based upon the dominant sub-species inherited from their lineage, for example, pure indica, mostly indica, mostly sativa, or pure sativa. Instead of using pure indica or pure sativa, many patients can benefit from the use of hybrid strains. There are a vast number of strains available for patients, each with a different cannabinoid profile and effect. The genetics and hence the effects of one lineage will usually be dominant. For example, indica-dominant crosses are for pain relief, with the sativa component helping with energy and activity levels. Sativa-dominant crosses are good for stimulating appetite, with the indica component helping to reduce body pain and increase relaxation.

The efficacy of cannabis is directly related to strain selection. Care should be taken when selecting strains that will benefit you. Potency and dosage vary with different strains, conditions, and individuals. The idea is to consume as little as possible of the most appropiately potent strains available in order to reduce costs and potential side effects.

There are approximately 60 identified cannabinoids and each of an infinite number of strains of cannabis has its own cannabinoid profile. The active cannabinoids each have unique physiological effects and many combinations actually appear to have synergystic and antagonistic effects.

CONCLUSION

In light of this information about cannabis and its extracts, its relatively low toxicity and emerging benefits, what I personally recommend is to work with your doctor or naturopath to determine which type of cannabis would best meet your needs, and then some trial and error will be required to adjust dosages. Your cannabis dispensary, if legal in your state, can also be helpful in providing you information on the strains available. Of course I am also available for personal consultation.

6.

Transdermal and Oral Cannabis

Although medical marijuana is nontoxic, smoking it can be hazardous over the long-term because toxic compounds are created in the combustion process. Fortunately there are options for the administration of cannabis, but in general all different ways of administrating hemp oil or raw marijuana can be combined with no harmful side effects. Also there are vaporizers that allow for inhalation or what amounts to transdermal treatments into the lungs without burning the marijuana. It's a cool clean smoke of powerful medicine.

SMOKING MEDICAL MARIJUANA

Smoking marijuana has limited medical value when used exclusively, especially when it is inhaled through burning. It can reduce blood sugar; it can also help reduce ocular pressure for people with glaucoma. Most people know of marijuana's ability to reduce nausea, and smoking marijuana will often reduce the pain associated with many medical conditions. Smoking "grass" does make a person relax, which in itself can be quite beneficial. Smoking does help reduce the symptoms of many conditions, but in general it does not work on a curative level like oral consumption does.

Rick Simpson, the most courageous medical marijuana expert of them all, says, "Smoking is the least effective method of using hemp as a medicine. The power of hemp medicine is magnified many times when the concentrated essential oil of the hemp plant is produced. If you want to see the real medicinal magic in the hemp plant, start ingesting high-grade hemp oil. When one starts ingesting the raw, unburned THC and its associated cannabinoids, medical miracles often occur. When a person smokes a joint, over 90 percent of the medicinal aspect of the plant material goes up in smoke. It's ironic to see people who have taken chemotherapy smoke hemp to reduce their nausea. They are smoking the very substance that, if taken properly, could cure them."

ORAL MARIJUANA

Cannabis, or marijuana, has been utilized as an ingredient in food and drink for thousands of years. Recipes were often recorded in rhyme, assisting in the memorization process. One such recipe, Bhang (a milk-based drink), dates back to 800 B.C. when it was first concocted in India. The Chinese use of cannabis as a staple food source—for both humans and animals—dates back to the 7th century B.C. Gathered for their exceptional nutritional value, cannabis seeds provided an exceptional source of protein and nutrients.

When we ingest marijuana it is absorbed via the intestines and then passes through the liver, which processes the THC into a byproduct called 11-hydroxy-THC, which then travels to the bloodstream and then on to our brains. 11-hydroxy THC is thought to be four to five times more potent than regular THC. This is one reason why edibles are known to be more potent when compared to inhaled cannabis. Edibles are also thought to be strong sedatives and many patients use them for treatment of insomnia. Marijuana taken in edible form usually takes from 40 minutes to one hour to start working and the peak effect is at two hours. The effects last though from 6 to 8 hours, which is very convenient for those patients who want to sleep or have longer control of pain.

The key to proper use of oral marijuana is to know how much to eat so as to get the best medicinal effect without taking too much. The general rule is, if you buy an edible product from a registered marijuana dispensary, cut the edible product into four pieces and eat one piece to start. Wait at least one hour. If you feel braver start with half (two pieces)! If you feel the effects of the medication, do not eat any more. If you do not feel the effects of the medication, you can eat another piece. There have been patients who unknowingly have ingested too much and have felt "too high," nausea, vomiting, and very groggy, so it's best to start out slow in the beginning. If you do not feel much at a full dose than try a dose and a half or even two doses.

It turns out that **unheated** raw cannabis juice provides 60 times more THCa (the medicine molecule) versus heated! The new discovery is: heating cannabis decarboxilates most of the THCa (the medicine molecule) to THC (the psychoactive molecule). A gram of **heated** cannabis provides only 10 mg of THCa, an uneffective dose, while a gram of **unheated** cannabis provides 600 mg of THCa, an effective dose. THC is not the cure, THCa seems to be the real medicinal in the plant. So, in summary **heated** cannabis (mostly THC with only a little bit of THCa) helps heal, but **unheated** cannabis (60 times more THCa) helps heal 60 times more effectively! Sixty times better.

Raw Cannabis

In California an adult may grow, buy and smoke marijuana, all while remaining safely within the confines of state law. Dr. William Courtney tells his patients "Don't smoke the stuff. Eat it!" It won't get you high eaten raw and juiced with a handful of carrots to cut the bitter taste, its leaves and buds may well offer an important contribution to getting people well.

Kristen P. summarized her return to nearly full health—after debilitating lupus, interstitial cystitis, rheumatoid arthritis, and 40 medications a day—by juicing fresh pot leaves over a 30-month period.

Raw bud has a high concentration of cannabinoids and is excellent for consumption. When consumed, raw marijuana generally does not make a person high. The main psychoactive compound in dried, aged cannabis is delta-9 THC, which is absent in the raw, fresh leaf. However, the other compounds, such as the terpenes, may have an effect on mood or energy levels. Raw leaf contains mainly THC *acid* (not THC) unless you are using a strain that is much higher in CBD. In that case, you will be getting some CBD from the leaf. Leaves are picked from a plant that is about three months of age. Buds should be at the state where the trichomes are fully present but not yet amber (for example, cloudy).

Some of the benefits of raw cannabis include:

There are more than 525 molecules found in raw cannabis, some with synergistic effects.

- Anti-anxiety
- Anti-diabetic
- Anti-inflammatory
- Anti-tumor/anti-cancer
- Antibacterial
- Antioxidant
- Antispasmodic
- Bone stimulation
- Immune modulating
- Neuroprotective
- Pain-relieving

"Active" Ingredients in Raw Cannabis:

- Cannabichromene (CBC)
- Cannabidiol (CBD)
- Cannabidivarin (CBDV)
- Cannabigerol (CBG)
- Cannabinol (CBN)
- CBD Acid
- Flavonoids
- Phytocannabinoids
- Terpenes
- THC Acid

According to Dr. Courtney it takes about 4 to 8 weeks before full clinical benefit is reached. It takes that long to fully saturate the fat tissue with phytocannabinoids. Phytocannabinoids are fat molecules that are stored in the adipose or fat tissue similar to the fat-soluble vitamins A, D, E and K. It appears that a wheat grass juicer is probably the best method of breaking up the cannabis plant cells. Mix with a minimal amount of organic fruit or vegetable juice—just enough to cut the bitter taste of the raw cannabis. Choose lower sugar juices to minimize your ingestion of simple sugars. Store leaves in a green bag in the refrigerator; do not rinse until immediately before using. Dr. Courtney recommends soaking leaves in water for five minutes before juicing. Use organic cannabis that does not have any pesticides applied at any point in its life cycle. Dr. Courtney recommends using ten large fan leaves per day in juice, salsa, pesto, and salad. If you have access to fresh bud he recommends one bud per day.

Cannabinoids and THCA are cleared rapidly from the blood, so frequent consumption of a small amount of juice is ideal. Split the juice into five parts for five divided doses per day.

TRANSDERMAL MARIJUANA

Marijuana is lipophilic, which means that it can be dissolved into a fat-soluble substance and then readily enters cell membranes. In other words, it can be effective when applied topically on the skin. Marijuana can be used transdermally to relieve pain from many conditions. Medical marijuana can be a balm, lotion, ointment, or rubbing alcohol solution. In the old days when people only had plants to use for medication, many patients would soak marijuana leaves in alcohol and apply them as a poultice to an arthritic or swollen joint.

Many substances pass easily through the skin and that is why transdermal medicine has been more popular in contemporary medicine. When it comes to marijuana's anti-inflammatory effect, people have experienced this process in action when applying marijuana to their skin. Patients with arthritis, muscle and joint pain can testify to the easing of the aches and pains they feel on a regular basis. Topical marijuana preparations usually provide only local relief and do not have effect on the brain, meaning there is usually no high. This is helpful for those times when marijuana use is inappropriate (like when you have to drive your car) and you still need pain relief! Topical preparations can be purchased or made at home.

Transdermal medicine is ideal for pain management as well as sports and pediatric medicine. In fact it is one of the best ways to administer medicines quickly and effectively. Transdermal methods of delivery are widely used because they allow the absorption of medicine directly through the skin. Gels, emulsion creams, sprays, and lip balm stick applicators are easy to use and are effective in getting medicine into the bloodstream quickly.

Traditional methods of administering medicine, such as tablets or capsules, get watered down and become much less effective due to stomach acids and digestive enzymes before they eventually get into the bloodstream. Bypassing the stomach and liver means a much greater percentage of the active ingredient goes straight into the bloodstream where it's needed. In many cases, transdermal methods are used to help avoid potential side effects, such as stomach upset or drowsiness. The full potential for transdermal medicine has not been explored by modern medicine though it has been practiced for thousands of years in hot springs around the world.

Of course the use of magnesium oil for these same effects is also recommended, and using topical magnesium and marijuana together in combination is excellent for difficult, stubborn pain. One of the main points for everyone to understand is that when we are thrust back to simpler lives, having access to versatile medicines without cost is important. If the governments would get off their people's backs, marijuana would be legal and virtually free because it's so easily grown.

> *It is highly regrettable that the deficiency of such an inexpensive, low-toxicity nutrient like magnesium results in diseases that cause incalculable suffering and expense throughout the world.*
>
> —DR. STEVEN JOHNSON

Bottom line, when it comes to pain medications that work on the source of pain and disease, there is nothing like magnesium chloride and nothing like cannabinoid medicine. Together they are the Batman-and-Robin superhero medical team for the world of pain, heavy emotional upset, and the general treatment of disease. Add sodium bicarbonate (baking soda) and iodine and you have a full medical team at your fingertips.

HEMP SALVES AND OILS

One hospital pathologist cut his finger during an autopsy; bacteria resistant to antibiotics infected the wound and it seemed that an amputation was going to be inevitable. Then someone had the idea to ask Professor Kabelik, who was known for his research on the medicinal use of cannabis, for help. He applied his hemp salve and two days later the wound was already healing and the amputation was avoided.

"There is no better treatment for severe burns than hemp oil. If the oil is applied to a burn within minutes, it takes the pain away and greatly accelerates the healing process. I have seen severe third-degree burns healed completely in eleven days with no scarring. If hospitals would use hemp oil in their burn units, human suffering could be greatly reduced. Hemp oil is a natural anesthetic and a natural antibiotic, so there is no sensible reason why it is not being used by the medical system in their burn units," says Rick Simpson.

Topical Solution Uses:

- Arthritis
- Burns
- Dry/chapped skin
- Eczema
- Headaches or migraines
- Insect bites
- Muscle soreness
- Pain
- Psoriasis
- Rashes
- Rheumatism
- Stiff neck
- Sunburns
- Swelling
- Tendonitis

OTHER POTENT SOLUTIONS

A keen interest for using medical marijuana for pets has evolved and many medical marijuana patients are happy to learn about tinctures of cannabis.

Medical Marijuana for Pets

A Seattle company is reportedly developing a medical marijuana patch for pets, calling it a "question of quality of life." Jim Alekson's Medical Marijuana Delivery Systems, LLC has patented the patch, called Tetracan, and says it could be used on dogs, cats, and even horses. The patch would be available for human use as well. According to Alekson, "Dogs suffer from the same maladies that humans do," and pets can suffer greatly from pain—everything from arthritis to cancer. He said that harsh pharmaceutical painkillers have proven harmful, sometimes fatal to animals.

Marijuana Tinctures

A tincture is an alcohol-based liquid mixture. It is like a concentrated extract. Currently there are tinctures of cannabis made with alcohol, oil, or glycerin. It is a very effective way to use medical cannabis. Tinctures are fast-acting and allow patients to drink their medication with none of the harmful effects of smoke or calories involved in edibles. For instructions on making your own alcohol- or glycerin-based tinctures *see* Resources on page 180.

Tincture dosages are typically 1 to 2 teaspoons dissolved in a cup of water. Or drops of the tincture are placed under the tongue (sublingually) and the medication passes through the blood vessels and enters the bloodstream. Most feel the onset of effects in about 5 to 15 minutes with the peak effect at about 30 minutes after taking the medication. For many patients, the effects are similar to inhaled cannabis.

Benefits of using a tincture of cannabis:

- Can be used discreetly
- Fast-acting
- No equipment except the bottle and the eyedropper
- No irritating smoke
- No smell

Patients who require quick relief of pain (for example, for migraine headaches) find that taking quick action is very helpful. Patients who are unhappy or uncomfortable with the smoking aspects of marijuana use also enjoy the tinctures. It is interesting to note that tinctures of cannabis were widely available around the mid 1800s.

CONCLUSION

There are a number of ways to administer medical marijuana, and one method may be more effective than another. Users need to choose the method best to treat their condition or disorder. As you have learned in this chapter, the effectiveness will vary with each method.

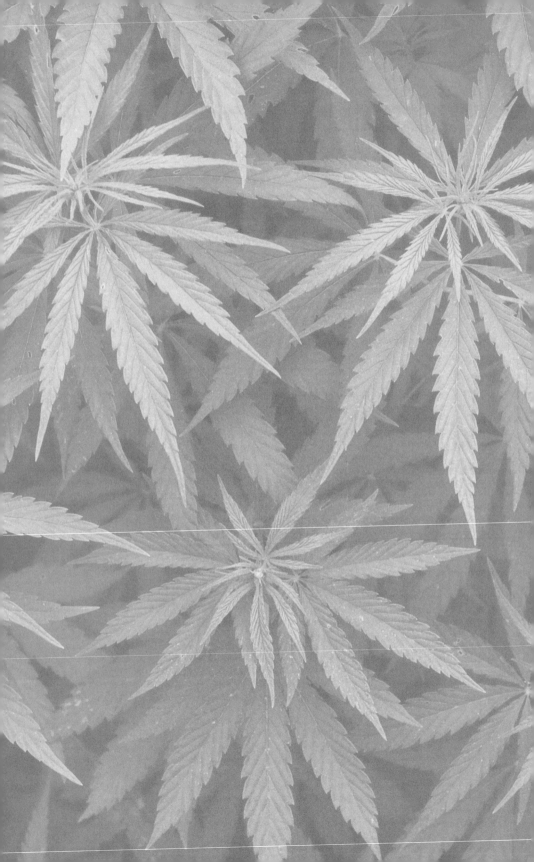

7.

Hemp Oil

Hemp seed oil is extracted from the seed of Cannabis sativa, commonly known as marijuana. The preparation used as a psychoactive drug (the highly publicized face of marijuana) actually uses the dried flowers and subtending leaves and stalks, not the seed. Versatile hemp seed oil has very low to undetectable levels of any of the psychoactive components called cannabinoids, making it safe to use in a variety of ways. The plant is also very hardy with a natural resistance to pests, which makes it an easy plant to grow organically without pesticides or herbicides.

The seeds of the plant are inclined to produce the best hemp oil, although the entire plant can be pressed for oil. Hemp seed oil has been called "Nature's most perfectly balanced oil." The latest science acknowledges that it contains all the essential amino acids and essential fatty acids (omega-3 and omega-6) fundamental for human life, as well as a rare protein known as globule edestins (a globulin legumin protein) that is akin to the globulin found in human blood plasma.

It is determined to be the optimum prerequisite for long-term healthy human nutrition. Research has shown that many common illnesses are linked to deficiencies or imbalances of specific fatty acids, such as omega-3, omega-6, and their derivatives. Hemp oil is also comprised of proteins which provide amino acids similar to the protein in meats and eggs. Cannabis seeds also contain a perfect balance of essential amino acids, B vitamins, calcium, magnesium, potassium, vitamin E, and carotene.

BENEFITS

As one of the world's most balanced and richest known sources of omega-3 and omega-6 fatty acids (EFAs), cannabis seeds are nutritional powerhouses. In the United States people are becoming educated in the benefits of hemp oil and the market for hemp seed oil is growing. An increasing number of people are seeking out the product for its reported health benefits. Hemp oil has a number of health benefits. The EFAs found in hemp seeds are known to have a number of health benefits and reduces the risk of:

- Anti-aging
- Arthritis
- Attention Deficit Disorder (ADD)
- Cancer
- Cardiovascular disease
- Diabetes
- Healthy hair
- Helps maintain hormonal balance
- Helps reduce the "bad" cholesterol
- Improves health of MS patients
- Nourish and moisturize the skin
- Osteoporosis
- Prevent depression
- Prevent skin disorders (psoriasis, eczema, acne, and dry skin)
- Proper organ function
- Ulcers

Although hemp oil has several health benefits, it should be avoided by prostate cancer patients and those who take blood thinners.

> *Ulcers within the body can be cured by ingesting the oil.*
> *Unhealthy ulcers, warts, and moles on the body can be*
> *removed by simply applying oil and covering with a bandage.*
> *The oil goes after unhealthy or mutating cells and*
> *destroys them painlessly in most cases.*
>
> —RICK SIMPSON

Rick Simpson, who uses hemp oil to cure cancer, says, "To treat internal cancers the oil must be ingested. I usually start people out with three or four doses a day, about the size of half a grain of dry rice. The only time I would suggest that people start with a heavier dose would be if there was a lot of pain involved with their condition. Oftentimes many of these folks are already addicted to dangerous and deadly pain medications. The object in such cases is to get these people off these dangerous drugs and to replace them with hemp oil to ease their pain. I suggest that about every four days the dosage be increased slowly until the patient has worked their way up to taking a gram a day. At this point most people continue taking a gram a day until they are cured. In more than one case I have seen people take the full 60-gram treatment and cure their cancer in a month."

Simpson continues, "We all have different tolerances for different med-ications so I encourage people to stay in their own comfort zone when dosing themselves with the oil. Most people's tolerances build very quickly and on average a normal person usually takes about 90 days to ingest the 60-gram treatment. Sixty grams seems to be able to cure most cancers, but people who have suffered extensive damage from chemo and radiation may require more to undo the damage the medical system has left behind.

It should also be mentioned that the oil rejuvenates vital organs like the pancreas. Many diabetics who have taken the oil find that after about six weeks on the oil that they no longer require insulin since their pancreas is again doing its job.

HOW TO USE HEMP OIL

Mixing hemp oil with facial creams does wonders for the complexion if you give yourself a facial with it; also, it should be used in such things as suntan lotions or some external skin conditions. Where full strength oil is not required, the oil can be mixed with skin creams and salves.

Rick Simpson says, "I always suggest to people that they ingest the oil for internal conditions. Often people come to me with lung cancer and other lung conditions. For such people I recommend the use of a vaporizer. Vapor-izing the oil along with ingesting it can have a very beneficial effect for those suffering from lung cancers. All they have to do is ingest their regular dose and take about two inhales from a vaporizer 2 to 3 times per day. By using this method the cancer is being attacked from both directions and this can greatly increase the effectiveness of the treatment. Herpes, skin cancer, warts, moles, and other skin conditions can be treated with pure oil with no allergic reactions. The only reaction I have witnessed with the use of the oil used top-ically was caused by the bandages used to cover it. When you use a bandage for extended periods it can cause the area covered with the sticky portion of the bandage to become irritated. One simply has to stop using the bandages for a day or two and the condition will disappear."

HEMP OIL HOME PRODUCTION

Rick Simpson recommends that "people grow their own hemp either in a small indoor grow system or outdoors. Growing it yourself will eliminate the high cost associated with buying hemp from drug dealers. The cost of hemp can vary greatly from dealer to dealer and so can the quality of the hemp." For anyone new to growing hemp, a good book or video on the subject is a necessity. If you go to Cannabis Culture, the good people there should be able to point you in the right direction.

Hemp Oil Cancer Dosage Information

By Rick Simpson

It takes the average person about 90 days to ingest the full 60-gram treatment. I suggest that patients start with 3 doses per day, about half the size of a grain of short grained dry rice. A dosage such as this would equal about 1/4 of a drop every eight hours. After four days at this dosage, increase your dosage to a half drop every eight hours and four days later increase the amount you are ingesting again to one drop every eight hours. The object is to try to double your dosage every four days, until you have reached the point that you are ingesting about nine drops of extract every eight hours and this amount would equal, about one-third of a gram or approximately one-third of a ml. Many patients will find this quite easy to accomplish, but those who have a very low tolerance may find it necessary to increase their dosage more slowly.

It takes the average person about 4 to 5 weeks to get to the point where they can ingest a gram per day. Once they reach this dosage they can continue at this rate until their cancer is eliminated. One gram is just slightly less than 1 ml, so either form of measurement works out to be about the same. For best results I believe that the extract should be taken early in the morning and then again in mid afternoon, and the last dosage of the day should be taken about an hour before bedtime. I must also mention the fact that many patients are able to ingest more than one gram per day and if they feel comfortable in doing so, this could help them deal with their medical problems much more quickly. In fact, I have received reports from some cancer patients who were deemed to be beyond hope with stage four cancers that took the full 60 gram treatment in one month, after which they were declared to be cancer free.

Using the method I have described allows the body to build up its tolerance slowly; in fact, I have received many reports from patients, who took the oil treatment and claimed they felt that they never even became high during the treatment. We all have different tolerances for any medication. Your size and body weight have little to do with your tolerance for cannabis extracts. Be aware when commencing treatment with these extracts that its effects will lower your blood pressure, so if you are currently taking blood pressure medication, it is very likely that you will no longer require its use. The same also holds true for diabetics, and many of those who suffer from this disease will find that their need for insulin will decrease very rapidly.

When people are taking these extracts, I like to see them stay within their own comfort zone, but the truth is, in a life threatening situation the faster you can take the oil, the better your chance of surviving. At the end of their treatment most people continue taking the oil but at a much reduced rate. I consider a good maintenance dose to be one or two drops at night, about an hour before bedtime, and this would mean that you are consuming 1 to 2 grams of high quality extract per month. I do not like to see patients overdosing on the oil, but an overdose does no harm and once patients become accustomed, to the effects these extracts can exhibit, many patients tend to enjoy the experience.

The main side effect of this medication is sleep and rest, which play an important role in the healing process. Usually, within an hour or so after taking a dose, the oil is telling you to lie down and relax. Don't fight the sleepy feeling, just lie down and go with it and have no fear, for you will not be harmed. Usually within a month, the daytime tiredness associated with this treatment fades away, but the patient continues to sleep very well at night. Once this takes place the patient can then safely drive their car again, since these extracts do not impair your motor skills and therefore, you will not present a hazard to others who are traveling on our highways.

The only time I would recommend that patients start out with larger doses, would be to enable them to discontinue the use of addictive and dangerous pain medications. When patients who are using such medications begin the oil treatment, they usually cut their pain medications in half. The objective is to take enough extract to relieve the pain and to help the patient get off these dangerous pharmaceutical medications as quickly as possible. Ingesting these extracts makes it much easier for the patient to discontinue the use of these harmful addictive medications, which the medical system employs, and properly produced cannabis extracts will greatly reduce their withdrawal symptoms.

I simply tell patients that the oil will do one of two things; it will either cure their cancer, or in cases where it is too late to affect a cure, the oil will ease their way out and they can at least then die with some dignity. Cannabis extracts have a very high success rate, in the treatment of cancer and most other diseases, but unfortunately many people who came to me had already been badly damaged from chemotherapy and radiation treatments. The damage such treatments cause have a lasting effect and people who have suffered the effects of these treatments are by far the hardest to cure.

> For those who have not allowed themselves to be damaged by chemotherapy or radiation the standard treatment is to ingest 60 grams of high quality extract over a 90 day period. But for those who have endured chemotherapy or radiation, I suggest that they should ingest 180 grams of extract to undo the damage these horrible treatments have left behind. It may take the patient six months to accomplish the task, but I feel that this will offer them the strongest possibility of making a full recovery.
>
> *Reprinted by permission of Rick Simpson [http://phoenixtears.ca/dosage-information/]*

I caution readers that oils that drug dealers sell can have many contaminants and often little or no THC. From my experience, most hemp oil available on the street should be avoided for medicinal use. Make your own oil (*see* page 56) or have someone you trust produce the oil to ensure that a very pure, high-quality oil is produced.

How much to make and take?

One pound (500 g) of bone-dry hemp buds will usually produce about 2 ounces (55 to 60 mL) of high-grade oil. This amount of oil will cure most serious cancers; the average person can ingest this amount in about three months. This oil is very potent so one must begin treatment with small doses. A drop of oil about half the size of a grain of rice, 2 to 4 times a day is a good beginning. After four or five days, start increasing your daily dosage very gradually. As time goes on the body builds a tolerance to the oil and more and more can be taken. In cases where people are in a great deal of pain, I recommend that their dosage be quickly increased until it kills the pain. High quality hemp oil will stop pain even when morphine is not effective. The oil can be applied to external injuries for pain relief in minutes.

Will I get high?

Following the dosage previously described, many people can take the full treatment and never get high. Even if a person does take too much oil the effect wears off quickly and no harm is done. No one has ever died from the use of hemp medicine.

Will I become addicted?

Hemp oil does not cause your body to crave more. It is non-addictive, harmless, and effective for practically any medical condition.

Is this the same as hemp seed oil?

No! This is hemp oil, made from the bud and small leaves of the hemp plant. It is the essential oil of the hemp plant. Health food store sells oil made from hemp seed that is often mislabeled as hemp oil. Although seed oil is very beneficial, it does not contain enough THC to have any effect on cancer and other serious illnesses.

Are hemp and marijuana the same?

The word marijuana is one of over four hundred slang terms used worldwide to describe the cannabis and/or the hemp plant.

Are all hemp plants the same?

When buying or growing hemp, procure a strain that has the highest possible THC content. To energize someone suffering from depression, I recommend a good Sativa strain. For most other medical conditions, I strongly suggest that Indica strains be used. Indicas relax a person and provide them with more rest and sleep.

How do I use it?

High quality hemp oil can be vaporized, ingested, or used topically. Add the oil to creams and salves for external use.

Where can I get information about making the oil?

For someone new to making the oil I suggest that you go to *Run from the Cure*. There you can watch our documentary in seven segments. Part 4 shows how the oil can be produced at home.

One can go to *Phoenix Tears Movie* and download the full documentary. You will need a high-speed internet connection and there is no charge. The process in the video could only be described as crude at best, but the oil that is produced will cure cancer.

In reality, this medicine should be produced in a controlled environment, using distilling equipment to reclaim the solvent and to purify the oil. Most people do not understand distilling and do not have access to the required equipment. This is the reason such a simple method is described in the documentary, so if need be, just about anyone can produce the oil. As in the video, again we stress that this process, if not done properly, can be dangerous and we bear no responsibility if this educational information is misused.

I am not a doctor and I do not have the right to tell people what they should do. Personally, I would not consider taking any cancer treatments currently

My Process

I generally work with a pound or more of good grade hemp starting material. You can use just one ounce. An ounce will usually produce 3 or 4 grams of oil. The amount of oil produced per ounce of hemp will vary from strain to strain, but it all has that wonderful healing power.

1. Place the completely dry starting material in a plastic bucket.

2. Dampen the material with the solvent you are using. Many solvents can be used. I like to use pure naphtha, but it costs $500 for a 45-gallon drum. You can use 99 percent isopropyl alcohol, which you can find in your local drug stores. Alcohol absorbs more chlorophyll from the plant material than naphtha does. This gives oils made with alcohol a darker color but does not diminish the potency of the oil to any noticeable degree. Ether, naphtha, or butane and many other solvents can produce oils that are amber and transparent. Granted these clear oils do look better but dark oil can be just as potent. If the process is done properly, little or no solvent residue is left in the oil. I have been consuming oils produced using different solvents for eight years with no harmful effects. You will require about two gallons of solvent to strip the THC off one pound of dry starting material; 500 milliliters of solvent should be more than enough to strip the THC from one ounce of hemp starting material.

3. Crush the plant material using a stick of clean untreated (chemical free) wood or some such device. Even though the starting material has been dampened with the solvent, you will find that the material can be readily crushed.

4. Add solvent until the starting material is completely covered. Use the stick to work the plant material. As you are doing this, the THC dissolves off the plant material into the solvent. Continue this process for about 3 minutes.

5. Pour the solvent-oil mix off the plant material into another bucket. You have just stripped the plant material of about 80 percent of its THC.

6. Second wash—again add solvent to the plant material and work it for another 3 minutes to get the other 20 percent.

7. Pour this solvent-oil mix into the bucket containing the first mix that was poured off previously.

8. Discard the twice-washed plant material.

9. Pour the solvent-oil mix through a coffee filter into a clean container.

10. Boil the solvent off. I have found that a rice cooker will do this boil off very nicely. The one I have has two heat settings—high and low—and will hold over a half gallon (2.5 liters) of solvent-oil mix.

11. Add solvent-oil mix to the rice cooker until it is about $^3/_4$ full. Make sure you are in a very well ventilated area and set up a fan to carry the solvent fumes away. The fumes are very flammable. Be sure to stay away from red-hot elements, sparks, and cigarettes that could ignite the fumes.

12. Plug the rice cooker in and set it on high heat.

13. Continue adding solvent-oil mix as the level in the rice cooker decreases until it is all in the cooker.

14. Add a few drops of water to the solvent-oil mix as the level comes down for the last time. The amount of water added depends on how much starting material you had in the beginning. If I am producing oil from a pound of good bud, I usually add about ten drops of water.

15. When there is about one inch of solvent-oil-water mix left in the cooker, put on your oven mitts, pick the unit up, and gently swirl the contents.

16. Continue swirling until the solvent has been evaporated off. The few drops of water help release the solvent residue and protect the oil some-what from too much heat. When the solvent has been boiled off, the cooker that I use automatically goes to low heat. This avoids any danger of overheating the oil. At no time should the temperature of the oil go over 290°F (140°C).

17. Put on your oven mitts and remove the pot containing the oil from the rice cooker.

18. Gently pour the oil into a small stainless steel container.

19. Place this container in a dehydrator or put it on a gentle heating device, such as a coffee warmer. It may take a few hours, but the water and volatile turpentine will be evaporated from the oil. When there is no longer any activity on the surface of the oil the medicine is ready for use.

20. Pour the hot oil into a bottle; or as in the video (*see* Resources on Page 180) suck it up into a plastic syringe. Putting the oil in a plastic syringe makes it very easy to dispense the medicine.

21. When the oil cools off it has the consistency of thick grease. Some strains will produce very thick oil, and you may have trouble squeezing it out of the syringe. If this happens, place the syringe in warm water a few minutes prior to use.

To anyone starting to use hemp oil as a medication, here are some simple facts. Hemp oil will lower blood pressure and if you are on blood pressure medication, you may find that this medication is no longer needed. The same is true for diabetics. I have seen hemp oil control blood sugar to the extent that insulin was no longer needed.

in use by our medical system; I do not recommend that hemp oil be taken along with chemotherapy. What would be the sense of making your own cure and then allowing the medical system to give you massive doses of poison?

From my experience with hemp medicine, I have found that most pharmaceutical medications are no longer needed once a person starts using hemp oil. Hemp oil seems to mix well with most natural medications, but I have had a few reports from people trying to take hemp oil and pharmaceuticals who experienced stomach pain. However, all problems ceased when they stopped taking the prescription drugs.

COOKING WITH HEMP OIL

Hemp seed oil is considered a super-food because of its high essential fatty acid (EFA) content, substances that we must ingest, since our bodies cannot make EFAs themselves. Cooking with cannabis need not be limited to medicinal uses. In addition to the number of ailments that cannabis can relieve, cooked marijuana is actually quite nutritious and can be incorporated proactively into your diet.

Refined hemp seed oil has primarily been used in body care products, but the unrefined oil has an attractive, nutty flavor, which makes it a great culinary alternative to other cooking oils. It contains highly digestible proteins and a quantity of trace minerals, making hemp seed oil one of the most nutritious food oils in use today. It's of particular use to vegetarians/vegans, as it provides a good source of alternative protein.

Combining marijuana with butter or oil is the most common way to cook with cannabis, but to get the benefits of hemp seeds many cannabis chefs choose to grind the seeds to produce a flour for breads, cakes, and cookies. If you want more ways to incorporate hemp seeds into your diet, you can also try incorporating hemp seed oil into your diet. As well as imparting foods with the many benefits discussed above, hemp seed lends foods a distinctive, nutty flavor perfect for adding depth and richness to any meal.

Hemp seed oil's light texture and unique flavor can accent and enhance a variety of foods, including salad dressings, pasta sauces, pizzas, hummus, and vegetable stir-fries. Care must be used during frying, however, since hemp seed oil has a relatively low smoke point. With proper precautions and a creative culinary mind, there is no end to the ways in which hemp seed oil can be used to produce unique, delicious dishes.

Making Ghee

Making pot ghee (a clarified butter) is fairly simple, but a bit time consuming (but nothing like making the hemp oil). You can start with butter, and make your own ghee, which is a process of putting butter in a pan, letting it melt, and then skimming off the solids as they rise up to the top. The solids are thrown away and what's left is ghee.

This ghee is then put into a crock pot/slow cooker, and the pot is put in with the ghee. The crockpot is kept on a medium/high temp for about four to six hours. Then the mix is strained with a metal strainer. The ghee should be green now. I take the pot that was strained out and put it in boiling water to get the last remnants of ghee to lift off of the pot, and then skim the ghee off of the surface of the water, and add it to the ghee mix.

I typically make enough at one time to fill a 32 oz container. This would be a couple of pounds of butter to start with. The ghee will be as potent as the pot that you put into it. A stronger pot equals a stronger ghee. I prefer it to be stronger, so I can use less of it in various recipes, and still get the desired effect. For storage, I keep the ghee in the freezer, but this is not essential. It can be kept unrefrigerated, just as regular ghee can be. (*See* website in Resources on page 180.)

Cooking with Cannabis Science—Cannabutter and Cannaoil

Cooking with cannabis is a precise process. Everything from heating temperature to solvent can affect the way cannabis will cook, and how it will affect the body. However, to understand the science of cooking with cannabis, it helps to have a basic understanding of the chemical compounds that make up the marijuana plant, as well as the ways in which these (and other) compounds are metabolized and digested by the human body when combined with foods.

Cannabis can be extracted into oils, such as olive oil or butter, for use in cooking, baking and salad dressings. Olive oil is a good choice of a healthy oil to use in this manner. The various ways to extract the THC in butter or oil can be found in the Chelsea Green blog, *see* Resources on page 180.

How to Make a Marijuana Topical Solution with Hemp Oil

If your state allows for medical marijuana dispensaries, you may be able to purchase topical solutions at these dispensaries. Otherwise, you may make your own by mixing hemp oil (using light almond oil or coconut oil is best) with beeswax or aloe vera.

Beeswax Balm

Mix 3 ounces of melted beeswax with 8 ounces of hemp oil. Cool and store in a sealed container in a dark cupboard.

Aloe Vera Lotion

Mix 8 ounces of aloe vera gel with 4 ounces of hemp oil. Store the mixture in a sealed container in the refrigerator.

SIDE EFFECTS

"The safety of this medicine is beyond belief. Even if a person overdoses badly there is no harm done to them once the effects of the oil wear off. The most common side effect we have noted with people ingesting hemp oil for their medical conditions is a great deal of rest and a smile on their faces. Yes, a person can get high if they take too much hemp oil, but if one uses common sense and starts with small doses, then gradually works their way up, in many cases 'getting high' can be completely avoided. I really don't understand why people would be concerned about getting high on the oil anyway since getting high presents no danger to them. They should be much more concerned about the effects of treatments like chemo. After all when you take enough poison to cause all your hair to fall out, that should tell you something," says Rick Simpson.

However, it does come with side effects, such as:

- **It's an Anticoagulant:** Hemp oil can have an anti-clotting effect on the blood. People who suffer from heart diseases and take blood thinners should avoid it (or at least check with a doctor before use!)

- **It Can Increase Prostate Cancer Risk:** Hemp oil has been shown to create the best conditions for the cells to regenerate, which could promote the growth of tumors, particularly prostate cancer cells. While more research is needed, medical professionals advise that you avoid consuming hemp oil if you are at an increased risk of prostate cancer.

- **In High Doses, It Could Cause Diarrhea or Cramps:** Large doses of hemp oil can cause nausea, diarrhea and/or abdominal cramps. For this reason, hemp oil should be kept out of the reach of children.

CONCLUSION

Hemp oil is an increasingly popular treatment product, and it is being used for a wide variety of purposes. Properly made hemp medicine is the greatest healer on this planet bar none. Once you experience what this medication can do, you will understand why history and I call hemp medicine a cure-all.

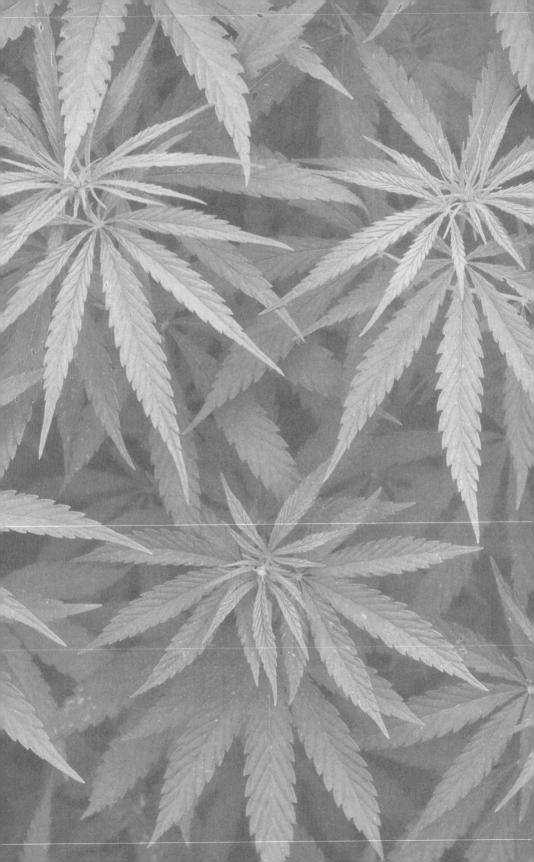

8.

The Law

Modern governments and contemporary civilization and medicine have conspired endlessly against the "reefer." Reefer madness—a term popularized by the 1936 movie *Reefer Madness*—is not something that is caused by smoking marijuana; it is something that came into being when certain industrialists turned the card-carrying members of society into marijuana haters and marijuana smokers into criminals.

The true crime against humanity is the dismissal of the great good this plant brings to men, women, and children. The war against drugs has been a cruel war conducted by people who believe in the rightness of their actions no matter how many lives they crush. This war has been a civilization-disrupting war and the powers that be have no intention of stopping. The rejection of marijuana as a potent medicine almost a century ago marked a strong movement into the headwinds of horrendous aggressiveness in allopathic medicine.

The DEA (Drug Enforcement Administration) Administrative Law Judge Francis Young declared in 1988 that medical cannabis is "one of the safest therapeutically-active substances known to man," but the government has continued to refute it. Doctors, in increasing numbers, are ignoring the federal government and are returning to a more natural form of medicine by electing to prescribe medical marijuana. This of course is happening only in the states where it has been made legal. The federal government still looks down on all of this with fiercely disapproving eyes, but the local natives don't pay them much attention, preferring to do what is right under state, not federal, law.

THE CAMPAIGN AGAINST MARIJUANA

Narcotics agents have terrorized anyone involved with marijuana. Millions have gone to jail; young people have lost college scholarships and had careers crushed; children have lost parents; families have disintegrated all because smoking a natural substance was prohibited and severely penalized. The war on drugs created misery for uncountable millions of people around the world in the 20th century and DEA agents are still at it.

> Jacob L. is a teenager facing life in prison for baking marijuana brownies in Round Rock, Texas. He is a high school student, who has never been in trouble with the law before, and is just the kind of kid that the federal government, police, and judges love to crush. Rapists love to attack women as these institutions love to attack and destroy the most innocent people you can imagine.

"In 2011, approximately 1,313,673 individuals have been arrested for drug-related offenses. Police arrested an estimated 858,408 persons for marijuana violations in 2009. Of those charged with marijuana violations, approximately 89 percent were charged with possession only. Moreover, since December 31, 1995, the U.S. prison population has grown an average of 43,266 inmates per year, with about 25 percent sentenced for drug law violations," wrote John W. Whitehead.

According to the FBI's Uniform Crime Reporting Program report, titled "2015 Crime in the United States," there were 1,488,707 total arrests for "drug abuse," a category that includes the sale, trafficking, and possession of drugs.

"The foot soldiers in the government's increasingly fanatical war on drugs, particularly marijuana, are state and local police officers dressed in SWAT gear and armed to the hilt. These SWAT teams carry out roughly 50,000 no-knock raids every year in search of illegal drugs and drug paraphernalia. As author and journalist Radley Balko reports, "The vast majority of these raids are to serve routine drug warrants, many times for crimes no more serious than possession of marijuana. . . Police have broken down doors, screamed obscenities, and held innocent people at gunpoint only to discover that what they thought were marijuana plants were really sunflowers, hibiscus, ragweed, tomatoes, or elderberry bushes," continued Whitehead.

THE MARIJUANA TAX ACT

The Marijuana Tax Act, which passed in 1937, coincidentally occurred just as the decoricator machine was invented. With this invention, hemp would have been able to take over competing industries almost instantaneously. William Hearst owned enormous acres of forest, so his interest in preventing the growth of hemp can be easily explained. Competition from hemp would have easily driven the Hearst paper-manufacturing company out of business and significantly lowered the value of his land.

DuPont's involvement in the anti-hemp campaign can also be understood in that they were patenting a new sulfuric acid process for producing wood-pulp paper. According to the company's own records, wood-pulp products ultimately accounted for more than 80 percent of all DuPont's railroad car loadings for the 50 years after the Marijuana Tax Act was passed.

Two years before the prohibitive hemp tax in 1937, DuPont developed nylon, which was a substitute for hemp rope. The year after the tax was passed DuPont came out with rayon, which would have been unable to compete with the strength of hemp fiber. DuPont's point man was Harry Anslinger, who was appointed to the FBN (Federal Bureau of Narcotics) by Treasury Secretary Andrew Mellon, who was also chairman of the Mellon Bank. Anslinger's relationship to Mellon wasn't just political, he was also married to Mellon's niece. The reasoning behind DuPont, Anslinger, and Hearst was not for any moral or health-related issues. They fought to prevent the growth of this new industry so they wouldn't lose money.

BIG PHARMA

Large pharmaceutical companies control the manufacture and dissemination of "legal" drugs in the world. *The Nation* published an interesting look at who's driving the fight against the legalization of marijuana. Pharmaceutical companies that make billions off painkillers and police unions are two big heavy hitters in the fight against marijuana legalization. They throw their monetary support behind groups that fight legislation that would legalize pot—even medical marijuana—and lobby Congress.

Millions of lives have been destroyed and uncountable millions suffer and even die because of the dangerous pharmaceuticals that are thrust upon the public in place of cannabis. This is a great wrong that needs to be made right and it can only be accomplished through full legalization.

> *The full therapeutic potential of cannabis can be realized only when it is completely legal and people don't have to go to their doctors to get it.*
>
> —DR. GRINSPOON

It is not the people who smoke marijuana who have suffered from Reefer Madness but the governments, police, and judges who en mass bent their minds and hearts to dark civilization disrupting ways.

No matter how much good there is to be found in the marijuana plant there will always be people who are against its legalization. Pharmaceutical giant Insys Therapeutics Inc., a manufacturer of fentanyl, just contributed $500,000 in the fight against marijuana legalization. This is one of the clearest examples of pharmaceutical terrorism that we can see. The company markets only this one product —a spray version of fentanyl, a powerful opiate.

Fentanyl is more potent than traditional addictive opiates, which already claim thousands of lives every year and drive addicts to graduate to heroin use. It is 50 times stronger than heroin and has been linked to a growing number of deaths in the United States. It is particularly dangerous when sold on the street and cut with other drugs. Fentanyl has been blamed for worsening the sharp rise in heroin overdoses as dealers across the country have begun adding it to heroin to make it stronger.

Yet Insys and opponents of legalization are more concerned about a plant. According to Arizonans for Responsible Drug Policy, "four states and the District of Columbia have already legalized [cannabis] and are seeing disastrous repercussions for their youth, workplaces, and communities." The drug war on people is alive and well even as legalization efforts continue to go through.

LEGALITY AND DOCTORS

A Las Vegas doctor who advocates medical marijuana therapy has been charged with illegally distributing prescription drugs. Federal agents arrested James Tinnell, 73. Tinnell said in 2005 that he had recommended medical marijuana to nearly 200 patients. On May 18, a federal grand jury charged Tinnell with 12 counts of unlawful distribution of controlled substances. Tinnell said he received his medical degree in 1962 from the University of Arkansas.

Dr. Allan Frankel has a lot of experience with the legal side of the marijuana issue. "In 2004, the United States Supreme Court upheld earlier federal court decisions that physicians have a fundamental Constitutional right to recommend medical cannabis to their patients. Within weeks of California voters legalizing medical cannabis in 1996, federal officials had threatened to revoke the prescribing privileges of any physicians who recommended cannabis to their patients for medical use. In response, a group of doctors and patients led by AIDS (Acquired Immune Deficiency Syndrome) specialist Dr. Marcus Conant filed suit against the government, contending that such a policy violates the First Amendment. The federal courts agreed at first the district level, then all the way through appeals to the Ninth Circuit and then the Supreme Court."

Frankel continues, "What doctors may and may not do. In Conant v. Walters, the Ninth Circuit Court of Appeals held that the federal government could neither punish nor threaten a physician merely for recommending the use of cannabis to a patient. But it remains illegal for a doctor to "aid and abet" a patient in obtaining cannabis. This means a physician may discuss the pros and cons of medical cannabis with any patient, and issue a written or oral recommendation to use cannabis without fear of legal reprisal. This is true regardless of whether the physician anticipates that the patient will, in turn, use this recommendation to obtain cannabis. What physicians may not do is actually prescribe or dispense cannabis to a patient or tell patients how to use a written recommendation to procure it from a cannabis club or dispensary. Doctors can tell patients they may be helped by cannabis. They can put that in writing. They just can't help patients obtain the cannabis itself."

"Patients are now protected. A December 2003 decision by a federal appeals court in Raich v. Ashcroft established that it is legal under federal law for patients to grow, possess, and consume medical cannabis, so long as they don't pay for it or cross state lines. The ruling applies directly to the nine western states in the Ninth Circuit's jurisdiction, but the precedent has been set for the nation. The federal prohibition on cannabis for any use does not apply to patients in these circumstances, and the federal government has been enjoined against arresting or prosecuting them."

High-ranking government officials in the United States have referred to the concept of medical marijuana as a hoax. One might ask why the government of the United States, the leading oppositional force to its legalization, clings so tenaciously to its insular and deplorable policy? Dr. Kate Scannell writes passionately about this issue saying, "I've seen one too many old men spend their final hours nauseated and vomiting while their distressed and helpless families watched… one too many women with cancer who linger, bone-thin and languid, as their loved ones beg for 'something' to make them feel better. And I, like so many doctors, have witnessed the therapeutic relief that many such patients experience after using marijuana. Their illnesses become less miserable, their difficult deaths are made more tolerable. And those reasons explain precisely why the federal government's relentless attempts to bar patients from access to medical marijuana constitute both cruel and unusual crimes against us all. They are wrong-headed and politically driven obsessions, not compassionate advisements intended to relieve human suffering."

CBD turns the debate about illicit-drugs-as-medicine on its head—medical marijuana that does not get the user high. One woman with Parkinson's disease, who treats, told him she ingests an oral marijuana candy, a medicine that does not make her intoxicated in order to calm her tremors enough so she can sleep. "She doesn't want to get high," said Dr. Callton (also a Michigan Republican Representative). "She just wants to sleep."

DECRIMINALIZING MARIJUANA

On one level little has changed since I first wrote the first edition of this book in 2010, central governments everywhere and most States in the U.S. still have draconian laws in place, but there is a large movement gaining steam on an international level of decriminalization.

However to see how much things are changing *The New York Times* editorial board recently endorsed the repeal of federal law banning marijuana. *The Times* argues that the ban on marijuana has caused "great harm on society just to prohibit a substance far less dangerous than alcohol. The social costs of the marijuana laws are vast. There were 658,000 arrests for marijuana possession in 2012, according to FBI figures, compared with 256,000 for cocaine, heroin, and their derivatives. Even worse, the result is racist, falling disproportionately on young black men, ruining their lives and creating new generations of career criminals. There is honest debate among scientists about the health effects of marijuana, but we believe that the evidence is overwhelming that addiction and dependence are relatively minor problems, especially compared with alcohol and tobacco. Moderate use of marijuana does not appear to pose a risk for otherwise healthy adults."

Is humanity coming to its senses or is there something sinister behind even the United Nations sponsoring the effort. A report published in July of 2014, by the World Health Organization, an agency of the United Nations, makes a discreet but clear call to decriminalize cannabis and even injecting drugs. There is a growing movement among scientific and political leaders to end the war on drugs entirely, however we can suspect that globalist elites triggered cannabis legalization for a variety of reasons.

The Daily Bell is suspicious of the motives behind the United Nations in this regard saying, "Global elites probably want to decriminalize drugs in order to provide the UN with the opportunity to regulate them; the idea is to reinforce an emergent, international licensing regime complete with global taxes and harmonized regulatory structure. In other words, the reason for drug legalization is not a beneficent one. It's all about yet more command and control. In a sense, it's disturbing because it amply indicates that the Western judicial system is mainly a play-thing of globalist priorities. Wars, prohibitions, and political structures all wax and wane in the modern era based on the power elite's internationalist agenda. Disturbing—yes. God knows how much blood has been shed over the "war on drugs," how many families have been ripped apart, how many lives have been ruined by incarceration and subsequent violence."

Rob Kampia, one of the movers and shakers in the decriminalization effort in the United States says, "Decriminalization is a step forward. It keeps marijuana users from being jailed and in some cases prevents them from being saddled with criminal records. But a more comprehensive solution is needed. Until we address how marijuana is being cultivated and sold, we will continue to see problems associated with prohibition. We will continue to see law enforcement officials waste their time arresting and prosecuting adults for marijuana offenses. We will continue to see marijuana sold in an oftentimes— violent underground market. And we will continue to have no real control over the product."

Even as marijuana becomes more popular, especially in medical and health circles, the campaign continues not only against users but also against researchers. A University of Arizona researcher hoping to explore whether marijuana can help veterans with post-traumatic stress disorder was fired in a move that she said was payback for her high-profile advocacy regarding the work.

In August of 2014 the *New England Journal of Medicine* wrote, "As Massachusetts prepares to implement its new medical-marijuana law, agents of the federal Drug Enforcement Administration (DEA) have reportedly visited at least seven Massachusetts physicians at their homes or offices and told them they must either give up their DEA registration or sever formal ties with proposed medical marijuana dispensaries. These encounters were meant to intimidate the physicians and to discourage them from taking an active role in medical marijuana dispensaries, and they have apparently succeeded.

MEDICAL MARIJAUNA EXISTS—SYNTHETIC KNOCKOFFS

According to the DEA medical marijuana already exists. It's called Marinol, which is widely available through prescription. It comes in the form of a pill and is also being studied by researchers for suitability via other delivery methods, such as an inhaler or patch. The active ingredient of Marinol is synthetic THC, which has been found to relieve the nausea and vomiting associated with chemotherapy for cancer patients and to assist with loss of appetite with AIDS patients. Radiation and chemotherapy often include violent, gut-wrenching nausea. Delta-9 THC is legally prescribed for counteracting the severe side effects of these cancer therapies, and is prescribed by doctors under its trade name, Marinol.

Marinol pills, which are taken orally to control vomiting, were shown to be a superior anti-emetic (anti-nausea) drug in six out of seven well-controlled studies reported in the *Journal of the American Medical Association* as early as 1981. However, Marinol falls short of perfection because of its super high potency, which often leads to intoxication and sedation. Also, oral administration is the least preferable method in this circumstance.

The paradox of swallowing a pill to eliminate vomiting has been noted by many physicians and patients as well as the American Medical Association. Ralph Seeley, an attorney who petitioned the State of Washington for access to medical cannabis and later died of bone cancer, was quick to point out,

"I don't know how many times I've taken one of those $12 pills and had it come right back up."

Marijuana is commonly smoked, which is a quicker and more effective method than oral administration. In the words of the National Cancer Institute, "Marijuana cigarettes have been used to treat chemotherapy-induced nausea and vomiting, and research has shown that THC is more quickly absorbed from marijuana smoke than from an oral preparation."

A careful study determining that marijuana is more effective than Marinol was published in 1988, but only one other research group, the Tennessee Board of Pharmacy, has been bold enough to confirm those findings. The National Institutes of Health is officially knowledgeable that smoked marijuana is more effective than Marinol tablets; panelists of the NIH Workshop on the Medical Utility of Marijuana in 1997 made very strong statements about marijuana's safety and medicinal value.

A report from the Brettler Center for Medical Research at Hebrew University in Jerusalem administered delta-8 THC, a non-psychoactive cannabinoid not found in the Marinol tablet, to eight children receiving chemotherapy treatments. Reportedly, "Vomiting was completely prevented." It is clear that the Marinol pill does not contain the complete range of medicinal cannabinoids shown to be effective in treating severe nausea. *Many patients agree that Marinol is less effective than whole marijuana, and many cancer specialists concur.*

Just about everyone knows that synthetic knockoffs of natural substances are never as effective or as safe as the original natural substance, but at least pharmaceutical companies can make money because the synthetic copies are patentable. The United States government obviously knows that cannabinoids are valuable medicines, but still they ruthlessly go after anyone who is dealing with the more natural and safe stuff.

Synthetic copies of natural substances rarely if ever maintain the same pharmacological effects as the original, and we know this to be especially true in the case of marijuana and the chemicals the pharmaceutical companies manufacture to simulate natural cannabinoids.

Sativex is another cannabinoid pharmaceutical that was developed as a mouth spray by the GW Pharmaceuticals in the U.K. for multiple sclerosis patients, who can use it to alleviate neuropathic pain, spasticity, overactive bladder, and other symptoms. Sativex is also being developed in Phase III trials as a potential treatment to alleviate pain due to cancer.

RULINGS

In a potentially crushing blow to the patients in many states with burgeoning medical marijuana industries, the IRS has ruled that dispensaries cannot deduct standard business expenses, such as payroll, security, or rent. The IRS ruling is based on an obscure portion of the tax code—section 280E—passed into law by Congress in 1982 at the height of Reagan administration's "war on drugs." The law, originally targeted at drug kingpins and cartels, bans any tax deductions related to "trafficking in controlled substances."

Although several major medical associations and 16 states and the District of Columbia have passed humane laws allowing medical use of marijuana, the federal government still considers it a Schedule I drug, the most restrictive category with the harshest penalties. As long as this is still in effect few will see the United States government as compassionate and caring about its own people or anyone else around the world. The news has spread rapidly through the cannabis community and is likely to have a chilling effect on medical marijuana dispensary businesses.

Some members of Congress have taken up the cause knowing as they do that cannabinoid medicine brings a lot of soothing comfort and relief to sufferers of many of the major diseases of our times. Representatives Pete Stark, D-California, Barney Frank, D-Massachusetts, and Jared Polis, D-Colorado, have introduced legislation to ensure the medical marijuana industry is treated like any other business. Two Republicans—Ron Paul and Gary Johnson—also support the legislation.

Marijuana became legal for recreational use in Washington State and Colorado in 2012, and three U.S. states, Massachusetts, Nevada, and California, legalized marijuana for recreational use in November of 2016.

Pot legalization supporters have argued for decades that prohibition has failed to curb pot use, and that the policy enriches drug cartels, hurts casual users and deprives governments of a potentially lucrative source of tax revenue. An October 2011 Gallup Poll that found a record 50 percent of Americans support legalizing marijuana use, up from 36 percent five years before.

The governors of Washington and Rhode Island are petitioning the federal government to reclassify marijuana as drug with medicinal uses so that it can be regulated outside the jurisdiction of federal authorities. Of course, they are not the only states that are taking the decriminalization (and even legalization) of marijuana very seriously.

Michigan is one of 28 states where medical marijuana was declared legal by voters, yet the Attorney General of Michigan, Bill Schuette, in 2008 waged a war on the law and tried to limit when, where, and to whom it can be sold. The state's war on the medical marijuana law (that voters overwhelmingly passed by 61 percent) is so unpopular with the public that a movement to get marijuana fully legalized has begun there. More than 322,600 signatures from registered voters are needed to put the issue on the ballot during the presidential election.

Medical marijuana use has surged in the 15 states that allow its use. But in a decision announced on July 8th of 2011 the federal government ruled that marijuana has no accepted medical use and should remain classified as a dangerous drug like heroin. The decision, which comes just after the Obama administration announced that it would not tolerate large-scale commercial marijuana cultivation, clearly shows how against its own people the federal government can be. One way or another the federal government and the people who control it are determined to crush the use of marijuana so they can then let the pharmaceutical companies continue to hurt and kill hundreds of thousands of people each year.

DEA Administrator Michele M. Leonhart rejected federal approval of the humane use of marijuana to treat medical conditions because marijuana "has a high potential for abuse," "has no currently accepted medical use in treatment in the United States" and "lacks accepted safety for use under medical supervision."

Before the government made marijuana illegal, the American Medical Association disagreed with the DEA and very much accepted marijuana as a useful medicine. The federal government has acted as a many-headed beast that has set itself against the natural world. The present position of the federal government is destructive to society and the constiutition of the United States and beside the point it is stupid and does not make any sense.

A recent AMA report entitled, "Use of Cannabis for Medicinal Purposes," affirmed the potential therapeutic benefits of marijuana and called for more research. The report concluded that, "short term controlled trials indicate that smoked cannabis reduces neuropathic pain, improves appetite and caloric intake especially in patients with reduced muscle mass, and may relieve spasticity and pain in patients with multiple sclerosis." The AMA is the largest physician-based group in the United States and this report overturns their viewpoint adopted only eight years ago calling for maintaining marijuana as a Schedule I substance. The AMA maintains that the cannabis sativa plant (marijuana) contains more than 60 unique structurally related chemicals.

Despite much public interest, fewer than 20 small, randomized, controlled trials of smoked marijuana, involving about 300 patients total, have been conducted during the past 35 years (excluding trials of the chemical THC and synthetic analogs). The limited findings suggest that the government has not wanted to find one of the key answers to cancer, which marijuana extracts, or hemp oil, certainly is—a medically rational answer to cancer.

Of approximately 6,000 Israelis currently being treated with cannabis, most suffer from chronic pain and terminal illnesses. The therapeutic potential of cannabis has been known for many years and is recognized by the Health Ministry. "My life changed completely. My face went back to what it was, I lost weight, I became a human being again. People are afraid, but there are problems caused by taking so many medicines that it's hard to know what a person is suffering from. In the meantime, I am with marijuana. Dr. Baruch left me with one psychiatric drug, which he says is keeping me in balance for now, and he will gradually lower its dosage. I went down from 17 medicines to five, including those against pains, against the nerve damage in my hand and against heartburn," writes Sherwood from Israel.

The medical marijuana story is important for it is a story that planted the seeds for the destruction of society through the criminalization of something good. Marijuana is goodness itself in plant form, and as a medicine it offers exceptional healing horsepower for a wide variety of diseases and medical conditions. Through the defamation of its goodness, unfortunately we get to see the badness and ugliness of corporate-controlled medicine. "It is amazing that for my post-trauma I easily—and without unnecessary arguments—get hard drugs such as opiates. I call it medical heroin, because there isn't much difference between the heroin that's sold on the street and the OxyContin that is prescribed for me. I also get sleeping pills from the benzaprine family, and for dessert I am offered Ritalin. The paradox is that all these medicines are far more dangerous and addictive than marijuana," writes one patient.

It was an insane civilization-disrupting idea to make marijuana illegal. This means that the guys at the very top of the human heap who pull the strings hardest on those below them are pathological enough to cause a mountain range of pain. These people are deranged, believing that nuclear weapons and nuclear power plants are safer to have around in our civilization than a legally blessed plant medicinal famous for thousands of years of safe medicinal use. It is ridiculous to make drugs of any type into criminal acts when consumed. Drug problems belong to the area of health, medicine and psychology. When a human being abuses and becomes dependent on anything, it is not the role of the law; it is the duty of healthcare workers to help those who need and are interested in being helped.

After 40 years, the United States' war on drugs has cost $1 trillion and hundreds of thousands of lives, and for what? Drug use is rampant and violence even more brutal and widespread. Even U.S. drug czar Gil Kerlikowske concedes the strategy hasn't worked saying, "Forty years later, the concern about drugs and drug problems is, if anything, magnified, intensified."

For much of the past three decades, authorities have waged war against the importation and sale of marijuana and other illegal drugs. Billions of dollars have been spent on law enforcement and drug rehabilitation programs and millions have been thrown in jail. And now after all of this, many experts believe the widespread use and abuse of *legally prescribed* opioid-based drugs is creating a new and even more devastating drug epidemic.

MEDICAL MARIJUANA

The *Associated Press* wrote, "For the past three decades, Uncle Sam has been providing a handful of patients with some of the highest grade marijuana around. The program grew out of a 1976 court settlement that created the country's first legal pot smoker. Advocates for legalizing marijuana or treating it as a medicine say the program is a glaring contradiction in the nation's 40-year war on drugs—maintaining the federal ban on pot while at the same time supplying it.

One of the recipients is Elvy Musikka, the chatty Oregon woman. A vocal marijuana advocate, Musikka relies on the pot to keep her glaucoma under control. She entered the program in 1988, and said that her experience with marijuana is proof that it works as a medicine. They "won't acknowledge the fact that I do not have even one aspirin in this house," she said, leaning back on her couch, glass bong cradled in her hand. "I have no pain."

In 1976, a federal judge ruled that the Food and Drug Administration must provide Robert Randall of Washington, D.C. with marijuana because of his glaucoma—no other drug could effectively combat his condition. Randall became the nation's first legal pot smoker since the drug's prohibition."

Big Pharma Now Wants In

David Edwards wrote, "Just as the federal government is clamping down on medical marijuana dispensaries, the Federal Drug Administration (FDA) may be set to give Big Pharma the clearance to take over the market. In 2007, GW Pharmaceuticals announced that it partnered with Otsuka to bring "Sativex"—or liquefied marijuana—to the U.S. The companies recently completed Phase II efficacy and safety trials testing and began discussion with the FDA for Phase III testing. Phase III is generally thought to be the final step before the drug can be marketed in the U.S. Sativex is the brandname for a drug derived from cannabis sativa. It's an extract from the whole plant cannabis, not a synthetic compound.

CONCLUSION

Dr. Carter has these closing words: "Physicians must take special care when discussing medicinal marijuana with their patients and be sure they understand the state and local laws governing what physicians can safely say and what patients can legally possess and use. As with any medication, proper documentation of the risks and benefits and any other requirements mandated by local laws must be clearly noted in the medical record. Physicians must be careful not to let their enthusiasm, frustration, and concern for suffering cause them to be careless when taking advantage of any law allowing their patients to use medicinal marijuana. Physicians who frequently authorize the therapeutic use of marijuana could potentially be investigated by authorities for compliance with the law, even in the form of an undercover agent disguised as a patient.

Fortunately, despite threats from former "drug czar" Barry McCaffrey and former Attorney General Janet Reno, no physician has yet lost his or her license to prescribe medications or has been prosecuted federally for authorizing the medicinal use of marijuana. At the state level, compliance with the terms of the local law allowing medicinal use of marijuana continues to protect the physician who authorizes such use to alleviate suffering."

In a toxic world, the antioxidant effects of marijuana might make it a required medicinal for survival in the 21st century.

The tide has turned in favor of legalization of marijuana for both medical and recreational purposes.

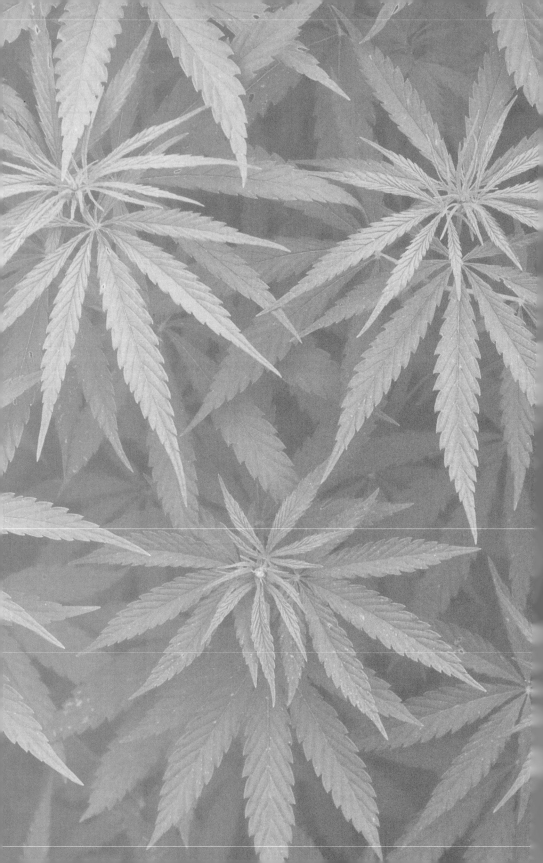

PART 2

TREATING HEALTH CONDITIONS

An Alphabetical Guide to Using Medical Marijuana

Cannabinoids reduce inflammation in the brain and prevent cognitive decline. Cannabinoids have also been shown to alleviate neuropathic pain. The THC molecule can directly impact Alzheimer's disease pathology as well as that for Parkinson's, autism, and all other neurological disorders. Maria L. de Ceballos, PhD, group leader in the Department of Neural Plasticity at the Cajal Institute in Spain, wrote, *"Our results indicate that cannabinoid receptors are important in the pathology of* Alzheimer's disease *and that cannabinoids succeed in preventing the neurodegenerative process occurring in the disease."*

Cannabinoids have been shown to modulate a variety of immune cell functions in humans and animals and more recently, have been shown to modulate T-helper cell development, chemotaxis, and tumor development. Many of these drug effects occur through cannabinoid receptor signaling mechanisms and the modulation of cytokines and other gene products. It appears the immunecannabinoid system is involved in regulating the brain-immune axis and might be exploited in future therapies for chronic diseases and immune deficiency.

Nausea appetite loss, pain and anxiety are all afflictions of wasting, and all can be mitigated by marijuana.
—INSTITUTE OF MEDICINE (IOM)

In *The Healing Brain,* a book by Dr. Robert Ornstein we see the brain not solely as an organ of rational thought but also as a gland. The brain is not just an organ used for thinking; it is a vast chemical manufacturing complex, producing many potent hormones and neurotransmitters that have strong effects on our psychological and physiological health. Certain brain neurotransmitters have antidepressant and anti-anxiety effects and regulate appetite. The neurotransmitter released by the postganglionic neurons is noradrenaline (also called norepinephrine). The release of noradrenaline stimulates heartbeat, raises blood pressure, dilates the pupils and shunts blood away from the skin and viscera to the skeletal muscles, brain, and heart while it inhibits peristalsis in the gastrointestinal (GI) tract. In short, stimulation of the sympathetic branch of the autonomic nervous system prepares the body for emergencies, for the "fight or flight" response.

CB1 receptors and ligands are found in the brain as well as immune and other peripheral tissues. Conversely, CB2 receptors and ligands are found primarily in the periphery, especially in immune cells. Cannabinoid receptors are G protein-coupled receptors, and they have been linked to signaling pathways and gene activities in common with this receptor family.

Dr. Gregory Carter says, "The cannabinoid system appears to be intricately

What we found is old animals have the receptors, and they actually get better if we treat them with the drug. If we give an old rat a high enough dose . . . we will reduce their brain inflammation and what we actually do is make them smarter as we do it.

—Dr. Gary L. Wenk, Professor of Psychology, Ohio State University

involved in normal human physiology, specifically in the control of movement, pain, memory, and appetite among others. Widespread cannabinoid receptors have been discovered in the brain and peripheral tissues. The cannabinoid system represents a previously unrecognized ubiquitous network in the nervous system. There is a dense receptor concentration in the cerebellum, basal ganglia, and hippocampus, accounting for the effects on motor tone, coordination, and mood state. There are very few cannabinoid receptors in the brainstem, which may explain marijuana's remarkably low toxicity.

Pesticides can cause brain damage and trigger conditions such as epilepsy, multiple sclerosis, and Parkinson's disease, according to scientists. A new landmark study claims that chemicals routinely used by farmers in the U.K. and around the world can result in neurological diseases. The controversial findings will be challenged by the agro-chemical industry, of course, who continue to insist that exposure levels for humans are well within safety limits. Greenpeace sponsored a study in India that also found large neurological consequences to pesticides, which are, after all, designed to kill. The largest basic assumption throughout the world of allopathic medicine is that all chemical exposures are within safety limits. Thus doctors are not prepared to address multiple toxic insults and the treatment for them.

Excessive levels of non-essential toxic elements, such as lead, cadmium, mercury, and aluminum have an "unbalancing" effect on essential trace element balances in the body's cells.

The following list of conditions covers a wide range of disorders, but it is, by no means, comprehensive of what can be treated through the use of medical marijuana. Included for each condition are the symptoms, triggers, the suggested conventional medications and their side effects, the benefits of medical marijuana, and lastly how medical marijuana alleviates the symptoms without adverse effects.

It is important to note that if you suffer from COPD (chronic obstructive pulmonary disease) or any lung disorder, smoking medical marijuana may cause harm and result in adverse consequences. It is therefore recommended to use medical marijuana compounds in other forms when needed.

AIDS

See **CANCER.**

ALLERGIES

Allergies occur when your immune system reacts to a foreign substance which may not cause a reaction in most people. Your immune system produces antibodies that identify these foreign substances that inflame your sinuses, digestive system, airways, or skin. Allergies can occur in various forms, such as food allergies, skin allergies, dust and mold allergies, pet allergies, allergies resulting from insect stings, eye allergies, drug allergies, allergic rhinitis, and latex allergies.

Symptoms

Allergy symptoms surface when your immune system reacts to an allergen or triggers. Exposure to these allergens may result in a variety of symptoms, including:

- Anaphylaxis (can be life-threatening)
- Diarrhea
- Headache
- Nausea
- Runny nose
- Skin rash
- Sneezing
- Swelling

Triggers

The most common culprits or allergens that can cause an adverse reaction are:

- Drugs
- Dust
- Foods (such as eggs, milk, peanuts, tree nuts, fish, shellfish, wheat, and soy)
- Insect stings
- Latex
- Mold
- Pets
- Pollen
- Ragweed

Benefits

Cannabis skin lotions have been shown to be effective in treating eczema. The Mayo Clinic discloses that cannabis or hemp seed oil has been found effectual for treating atopic dermatitis. Allergies are the most common cause of asthma and cannabis has been proven to reduce inflammation and relax constricted muscles in the airways.

Conventional Medicine

Over-the-counter and prescription drugs are usually prescribed to ease the symptoms associated with allergies, such as antihistamines, decongestants, and steroids. These medications may exhibit several adverse side effects. For instance, antihistamines may cause drowsiness, dizziness, confusion, and blurred vision. Potential side effects of oral decongestants may include a fast heartbeat, high blood pressure, and dizziness. Steroids carry a risk of side effects as well. The side effects may include elevated pressure in the eyes (glaucoma), high blood pressure, fluid retention, moodiness, and weight gain.

Medical marijuana

Cannabis can help in the treatment of allergies and autoimmune disorders that occur when body tissues are attacked by its own immune system. Extracts of the hemp plant cannabis are traditionally used as a popular remedy against inflammation.

See also **INFLAMMATION.**

ALZHEIMER'S

Alzheimer's disease is an illness of the brain. It causes large numbers of nerve cells in the brain to die. This affects your ability to remember things and think clearly. Doctors don't know what causes the disease. They do know that it usually begins after age 60 and nearly half of people age 85 and older may have Alzheimer's. However, it is not a normal part of aging. This neurological disorder is characterized by not only a progressive loss of memory but learned behavior as well.

Symptoms

Patients with Alzheimer's are also likely to experience depression, agitation, and appetite loss, among other symptoms. A chronic, progressively worsening problem can occur accompanied by:

- Concentration, lack of
- Disorientation
- Dramatic personality changes

- Eventually the loss of the ability to perform basic self-care functions
- Language and mathematical skills, lack of
- Problems with physical coordination
- Problems with judgment
- Repetition of the same ideas or movements
- Sleeplessness
- "Sunsetting" or restlessness (wandering off in the late afternoon and night)
- Tendency to wander off and get lost

Over 4.5 million Americans are estimated to be afflicted with the disease. No approved treatments or medications are available to stop the progression of Alzheimer's, and few pharmaceuticals have been FDA-approved to treat symptoms of the disease.

> *Alzheimer's disease (AD) is the number 4 killer of Americans, causing over 100,000 deaths each year in the USA alone. More than half of nursing home beds are occupied by AD patients.*

Triggers

Brain inflammation contributes to many age-related degenerative brain disorders, including Alzheimer's disease. "Inflammation appears to be present many, many years prior to the onset of the symptoms," says Dr. Gary L. Wenk from Ohio State University. Dr. Wenk and his associates have discovered that daily treatment with cannabinoids reduced inflammation in the brain and improved memory. Studies have shown that people who routinely use anti-inflammatory drugs, particularly the ones that cross the blood brain barrier, have a significantly reduced incidence of Alzheimer's disease. *Marijuana has strong anti-inflammatory effects.* "This is why I believe that people who used marijuana a few decades ago are much less likely to develop any disease, such as Alzheimer's, that relies upon the slow development of brain inflammation," said Wenk.

Undoubtedly the trigger mechanism of Alzheimer's is the accumulation of heavy metals in the nervous system causing free radical damage leading to DNA and mitochondrial DNA (mtDNA) damage. Yet according to the current level of medical science, most cases of Alzheimer's disease cannot be diagnosed with 100 percent certainty until a brain autopsy has been performed after death. The first half of the etiology of Alzheimer's disease is an increased profile of heavy metals, specifically mercury and aluminum and other toxic chemicals, especially pesticides that are designed to destroy the life forms they encounter.

Aluminum. Autopsy reports on Alzheimer's patients found 70 percent more aluminum in the brain. Aluminum is extremely harmful to life. Aluminum is a protoplasmic poison and a deadly, persistent neurotoxin. Aluminum can cause encephalitis, bone disease, and anemia in susceptible people. Though aluminum is less toxic than mercury, arsenic, lead or cadmium, it is a persistent poison that increases the toxicity of other heavy metals.

Dr. Chris Shaw found in animal studies that aluminum hydroxide shows statistically significant increases in anxiety (38 percent); memory deficits (41 times the errors as in the sample group); and an allergic skin reaction (20 percent). Tissue samples after the mice were "sacrificed" showed neurological cells were dying. Inside the mice's brains, in an area that controls movement, 35 percent of the cells were destroying themselves. Dr. Shaw shows a link between the aluminum hydroxide used in vaccines, and symptoms associated with Parkinson's, amyotrophic lateral sclerosis, and Alzheimer's.

Since 1934, aluminum hydroxide has been used as an adjuvant to boost the immune response from vaccines.

Mercury. Many researchers, with good reason, feel that the actual cause of Alzheimer's disease is due to toxic metal that leaches from mercury-silver amalgam dental fillings. Dr. Boyd Haley, a dental researcher from the University of Calgary, Canada, Dr. Murray Vimy, a member of the World Health Organization (WHO), and Dr. Fritz L. Lorscheider reasoned that because mercury vapor from amalgam fillings is absorbed into the sinuses and goes through the bloodstream directly to the brain, they might obtain stronger and more convincing results by exposing the rats in their experiments to mercury vapor.

The team calculated a dose of mercury vapor that would be the rat equivalent of humans inhaling the vapor from fillings. They exposed six rats to these carefully-measured quantities over a period of 7 to 24 days. The result was stunning: all six experimental animals treated with mercury vapor deteriorated markedly. When their tissues were examined, all six rats had brain aberrancies like those found in human Alzheimer's patients. In Dr. Haley's words, "The results of this experiment are terrifying. I'm getting the rest of my mercury fillings taken out right now, and I've asked my wife to have hers replaced too."

Dr. Haley reminds us that:

> In a human autopsy study, brain tissues from people with AD at death
> were compared with an age-matched group of control brains from sub-
> jects without AD. The only significant difference in metal content
> between the two groups of brains was mercury, being considerably
> higher in the AD group. Mercury concentration was prominent in the
> hippocampus, the amygdale, and particularly in the nucleus basalis, all
> brain structures involved in memory function. Dr. Fritz L. Lorscheider
> exposed a neuron in culture to 0.1 nanomolar mercury and filmed
> through a microscope. The result was that the axon broke open and the
> tubulin and tubulin associated proteins abnormally aggregated into a
> body that was "indistinguishable from a neurofibillary tangle" the sec-
> ond "diagnostic hallmark" of AD on pathology.

Clauberg and Joshi, in1993, have published in vitro evidence indicating
that aluminum may accelerate proteolytic processing of Aβ (amyloid-beta)
precursor protein by suppressing the inhibitory domain on proteolytic
inhibitors, thus contributing to the accumulation of Aβ.

In 1998 Julie Varner (INC Research) and two colleagues published
research on the effects of aluminum-fluoride and sodium-fluoride on the nervous system of rats. They concluded, "Chronic administration of aluminum-
fluoride and sodium-fluoride in the drinking water of rats resulted in distinct
morphological alterations of the brain, including the effects on neurons and
cerebrovasculature." Fluoride, lead, and aluminum together could be thought
of as a devil's triangle that acts not only to reinforce each other's toxicity but
also to greatly amplify the toxicity of mercury.

Flouride. "What is happening with Alzheimer's in the United States is not
typical of what is going on in the rest of the world," writes Lynn Landes, an
investigative reporter. "Americans account for 25 percent of all Alzheimer's
cases, even though we represent only 4.6 percent of the world's population.
Europe is experiencing half our rate of disease. For Americans over 85 years
of age, 50 percent are thought to have Alzheimer's. Fluoride is possibly the
missing link that greatly accelerates the progression of the disease. America's
drinking water is now over 60 percent fluoridated. Fluoride appears in many
processed foods and beverages made with fluoridated water. Keep in mind,
Europe has half our rate of Alzheimer's. They don't fluoridate their water
supplies, but they do use fluoride supplements and dental products."

Neurotoxic substances. Add to the formula the increased vulnerability of
neurological tissues and nerve synapses brought on by neurotoxic substances

like MSG and aspartame and we have the general diagnostic picture that health officials are incapable of understanding or appreciating. It is impossible for them, given their basic assumptions that all the following are safe: fluoride in dental products and drinking water, MSG, aspartame, mercury and aluminum in vaccines, mercury in dental amalgam, and the spreading pollution of mercury in the air, water, and foods we eat.

Dr. Russell Blaylock, neurosurgeon, speaking of the recent explosion in neurodegenerative diseases, says, "Things that used to be rare, we're seeing all the time now. It's just frightening. And when you look through the neurosciences literature, they have no explanation. They don't know why it's increasing so rapidly." This is ridiculous. They have no explanation for the disease because medical science is not interested in curing anything, as Dr. Alan Greenberg reminds us when he says, "Despite the investment of hundreds of billions of dollars of research, not even a single degenerative disease has been cured in the last hundred years."

Dr. Blaylock states clearly that the epidemic is here because we have such a large combination of toxins converging and simultaneously attacking the cells of our bodies. "For instance, we know that cellular neurodegenerative diseases are connected to mercury, aluminum, pesticides, and herbicides, and the way they produce brain damage is through an excitotoxic mechanism. So, we are all exposed to those toxins, and then when you add MSG and excitotoxins (aspartame) to the food, you tremendously accelerate this toxicity. That's why we're seeing this explosion in neurodegenerative diseases— Alzheimer's, autism, ADD, and Parkinson's—all these things are increasing so enormously because we are exposed to carcinogenic toxicity from all these different things along with this huge exposure to excitotoxins, which is the central mechanism," states Blaylock.

Magnesium deficieny. Massive magnesium deficiencies compromise cell health and physiological function on both sides of the blood-brain barrier. It's not just magnesium but a general malnutrition that accelerates the slide in neurological function. Magnesium though is the crucial nutrient/medicine that makes a big difference in prevention and treatment of Alzheimer's disease and associated disorders like ALS, Parkinson's, and the full range of autism spectrum disorders.

Although basic medical science already recognizes the dramatic physiological problem with widespread magnesium deficiencies, health and medical officials cannot form a basic conclusion about this and recommend magnesium treatments. They seem to be busy looking after their pharmaceutical financial interests, which would crumble if the truth about magnesium and the full dangers of medicine and dental products were ever made widely known.

Benefits

In older brains, but *not* younger brains, THC seems to have a protective effect. Campbell's findings (*Campbell Biology in Focus*) indicate that the biochemistry of neurons changes as the cells mature. The role of endocannabinoids shifts to regulate different functions—most important, assisting in the survival of aged neurons. In patients with Alzheimer's disease, THC protects neurons from death in several ways.

- THC boosts depleted levels of the neurotransmitter acetylcholine, which, when diminished, contributes to the weakened mental function in Alzheimer's patients.

- THC also suppresses the toxic effects of the so-called a-beta protein that may kill neurons in Alzheimer's disease.

- It stimulates secretion of neuron growth by promoting substances such as brain-derived neurotrophic factor.

- It dampens release of the excitatory neurotransmitter glutamate, which kills neurons by overstimulation.

- THC and other cannabinoids also have powerful anti-inflammatory and antioxidant actions that protect neurons from immune system attack.

Conventional Medicine

There are medicines that can treat the symptoms of Alzheimer's. However, there is no cure. Some medicines keep your memory loss and other symptoms from getting worse for a time. These medicines work best if Alzheimer's disease is found early. Other medicines work to help you sleep better or feel less worried and depressed. These medicines don't directly treat the disease. They do help you feel more comfortable.

The *New York Times* published an article about a study from the *New England Journal of Medicine* entitled "Alzheimer's Drugs Offer No Help, Study Finds." "The drugs most commonly used to soothe agitation and aggression in people with Alzheimer's disease are no more effective than placebos for most patients, and put them at risk of serious side effects, including confusion, sleepiness, and Parkinson's disease-like symptoms, researchers are reporting today." This was the third major study to cast doubt on the atypical antipsychotics, which were supposedly a significant advance over the first generation of antipsychotics.

Dr. Thomas R. Insel, director of the National Institute of Mental Health, said, "What this study shows is that these drugs are clearly not the answer; they may be helpful for a minority of patients, but we need to come up with better medications." Interestingly enough, another study revealed a natural medication that was much more effective and safer than the drugs most commonly used.

Prescription Alzheimer's drugs, such as donepezil (Aricept) and tacrine (Cognex) both work on the same enzyme-blocking principal. When researchers compared drugs to twice the concentration of THC, Aricept blocked plaque formation only 22 percent as well as THC. Cognex blocked plaque formation only 7 percent as well.

Medical Marijuana

New research from the Scripps Research Institute in La Jolla, California, reveals delta-9-tetrahydrocannabinol (THC), an active component in marijuana, can block the formation of brain clogging amyloid plaque in parts of the brain important for memory and cognition. Even more surprising, is that *THC's blocking power is more effective than some prescription Alzheimer's drugs.* The test-tube studies show that THC blocks an enzyme called acetylcholinesterase (AChE), which speeds the formation of amyloid plaque in the brain of people with Alzheimer's disease.

Dr. Kim Janda and colleagues used laboratory experiments to show that THC preserves brain levels of the key neurotransmitter acetylcholine. Janda's group reports in an article in the journal *Molecular Pharmaceutics*. Their experiments show that THC prevents formation of the amyloid plaques that are a hallmark of AD and its damage to the brain. Senescent (old) astrocytes are believed to be responsible for the production of the endogenous proteins, such as amyloid-beta protein (Aβ), that comprise the senile plaques that are fundamental to Alzheimer's disease.

> *THC is effective at blocking clumps of protein that can inhibit memory and cognition in Alzheimer's patients.*
> —JOURNAL OF MOLECULAR PHARMACEUTICS

The starting point for drastic changes in medical treatment of AD comes with the admission that present treatments are not safe or effective. The above studies leave us with no doubt that doctors are wasting more than time and money prescribing antipsychotics for the elderly. They are adding to their patient's toxic loads risking further complications and an earlier arrival of death.

Thus medicine has to take a serious look at what can be done to help the 4.5 million Americans who suffer from the progressive dementia of Alzheimer's disease. Alzheimer's is the leading cause of dementia among the elderly and the cost of caring for Alzheimer's patients is at least $100 billion annually, according to the National Institute of Aging. Alzheimer's cases are expected to triple over the next 50 years. Society and civilization itself is in desperate need for effective new treatments for Alzheimer's.

Investigators at the Scripps Research Institute in California in 2006 reported that THC inhibits the enzyme responsible for the aggregation of amyloid plaque—the primary marker for Alzheimer's disease—in a manner "considerably superior" to approved Alzheimer's drugs, such as donepezil and tacrine. "Our results provide a mechanism whereby the THC molecule can directly impact Alzheimer's disease pathology," researchers concluded. "THC and its analogues may provide an improved therapeutic [option] for Alzheimer's disease [by]. . . simultaneously treating both the symptoms and the progression of [the] disease."

> *THC can prevent an enzyme called acetylcholinesterase from accelerating the formation of "Alzheimer plaques" in the brain more effectively than commercially marketed drugs.*
> —SCRIPPS RESEARCH INSTITUTE IN CALIFORNIA

The amazing fact about the substance isolated from marijuana, which goes under the very prosaic title of WIN-55,212-2, is that not only does it reduce inflammation, it also stimulates the growth of new brain cells. Investigators at Ohio State University, Department of Psychology and Neuroscience, reported that older rats administered daily doses of WIN 55,212-2 for a period of three weeks performed significantly better than non-treated controls on a water-maze memory test. Writing in the journal *Neuroscience* in 2007, researchers reported that rats treated with the compound experienced a 50 percent improvement in memory and a 40 to 50 percent reduction in inflammation compared to controls.

> *Cannabis-based treatments could improve memory loss in Alzheimer's sufferers.*
> —ROYAL PHARMACEUTICAL SOCIETY OF GREAT BRITAIN

A cannabinoid is the signaling molecule within a unique system of communication that is intermittently activated between two of the brain's most ubiquitous nerve cells—neurons containing the inhibitory neurotransmitter

GABA and neurons containing the excitatory neurotransmitter glutamate. The modulation of inhibitory and excitatory signals leads to the regulation of excitation and inhibition within clusters of neurons that is the basis for all action and thought.

> *Signaling by the cannabinoid system represents a mechanism by which neurons can communicate backwards across synapses to modulate their inputs.*
>
> —Dr. Roger A. Nicol, UCSF professor of cellular
> and molecular pharmacology

Investigators at Ireland's Trinity College Institute of Neuroscience concluded: "Cannabinoids offer a multi-faceted approach for the treatment of Alzheimer's disease by providing neuroprotection and reducing neuroinflammation, whilst simultaneously supporting the brain's intrinsic repair mechanisms by augmenting neurotrophin expression and enhancing neurogenesis."

In the February 2005 issue of the *Journal of Neuroscience* researchers, who studied the brain tissue of deceased Alzheimer's patients, discovered that many of these patients lose the function of important cannabinoid brain receptors that seem to guard against cognitive decline. They further discovered in a rat study involving synthetic marijuana that when these brain receptors were working, they reduced the brain inflammation that is associated with Alzheimer's. "This is the first time the effects of such damage have been found in Alzheimer's patients," said study co-author Maria de Ceballos, head of the neurodegeneration group at the Cajal Institute, Spain's largest neuroscience research center in Madrid.

AMYOTROPHIC LATERAL SCLEROSIS (ALS)

Amyotrophic lateral sclerosis (ALS) also known as Lou Gehrig's disease, is a fatal neurodegenerative disorder that is characterized by the selective loss of motor neurons in the spinal cord, brain stem, and motor cortex. An estimated 30,000 Americans are living with ALS, which often arises spontaneously and afflicts otherwise healthy adults. More than half of ALS patients die within 2.5 years following the onset of symptoms.

Symptoms

The early symptoms of ALS can differ in one person to another. Typically ALS is a disease that includes a slow emergence. However, the rate at which the disease progresses can vary for different people. Painless, progressive muscle weakness is the typical primary symptom. Other initial symptoms vary, but can include:

- Abnormal fatigue of the arms and/or legs
- Difficulty chewing or swallowing
- Dropping things
- Muscle cramps and twitches

- Slurred speech
- Tripping
- Tight or stiff muscles
- Uncontrollable periods of laughing or crying

Seldom do people with ALS encounter similar symptoms or the same sequences or patterns develop. Though, continuous muscle weakness and paralysis are generally experienced.

Triggers

Evidence suggests that ALS may be triggered by exposure to heavy metals, pesticides, toxins, or fertilizers. It has also been suggested that a virus and strenuous physical labor or intense exertion may be responsible for the condition.

In 1907, Dr. Alois Alzheimer, a German psychiatrist and neuropathologist, first described a new ailment now known as Alzheimer's disease. Dr. Alzheimer's discovery occurred approximately 20 years after aluminum was introduced and became a widely used product. Dr. Michael A. Weiner, while doing research work in Japan, learned that Dr. Yoshira Yase had long held the opinion that aluminum may be a key player in amyotrophic lateral sclerosis (ALS). ALS is prevalent among the people on the Kii Peninsula of Japan and in certain groups on Guam. In many respects, ALS is similar to Alzheimer's. The soil and water in Guam and other areas in Japan where ALS is found, is high in aluminum and manganese and low in calcium and magnesium.

Benefits

Marijuana has now been shown to have strong antioxidative and neuroprotective effects, which may prolong neuronal cell survival.

Conventional Medicine

The drug riluzole (Rilutek) is the only medication approved by the Food and Drug Administration for treating ALS. It seems to slow the disease's development in some people. However, riluzole may cause side effects, such as dizziness, gastrointestinal conditions, and changes in liver function.

Medical Marijuana

Increasing amounts of evidence show that cannabis is a viable treatment option to relieve symptoms of ALS. The use of cannabis oil to treat ALS may actually prolong the life of the patient in addition to relieving many of the disease's devastating day-to-day symptoms.

In areas where it is legal to do so, Delaware, Washington, D.C., Georgia, Illinois, Maine, Massachusetts, Michigan, New Jersey, New Mexico, and New York, marijuana should be considered in the pharmacological management of ALS. Dr. Gregory T. Carter says, "Marijuana is a substance with many properties that may be applicable to the management of amyotrophic lateral sclerosis (ALS). These include analgesia, muscle relaxation, bronchodilation, saliva reduction, appetite stimulation, and sleep induction. Current scientific data (Carter et al., 2010) suggests that not only is cannabis significant in managing the symptoms associated with ALS, but it might notably slow the progression of the disease, potentially increasing life expectancy.

ANXIETY

See **EMOTIONAL DISTRESS, DEPRESSION, POST-TRAUMATIC STRESS DISORDERS, SLEEP DISORDERS, and STRESS.**

APNEA

See **SLEEP DISORDERS.**

APPETITE LOSS

Loss of appetite is when your desire to eat is reduced. It can be the result of a variety of disorders and diseases. Some can be temporary, such as a loss of appetite from the effects of medications, and some can be more serious, such as from the effects of cancer.

Symptoms

Related symptoms you may experience with a loss of appetite are weight loss and malnutrition. These conditions can be serious if left untreated.

Triggers

The loss of appetite may be triggered by a physical illness or condition or a mental condition.

Your appetite may decrease when you are experiencing sadness or stress, are grieving, or are anxious.

Certain physical or medical conditions may also cause your appetite to decrease, such as bacterial or viral infections, thyroid disorders, dementia, heart failure, hepatitis, HIV, chronic liver disease, or kidney failure. Cancer treatments, such as chemotherapy and radiation can also be a cause of appetite loss.

Certain prescribed medications and drugs may also decrease your appetite.

Benefits

Medical marijuana has been especially advantageous in alleviating nausea and stimulating the appetite, largely amongst the sick and among senior citizens who suffer from loss of appetite.

Conventional Medicine

The appetite-enhancing drugs most commonly prescribed include antidepressants, antiemetics (drugs prescribed for nausea and vomiting) and antihistamines. These types of medications can frequently cause a wide range of disagreeable side effects.

Medical Marijuana

Marijuana's well-known tendency to induce the "munchies" could potentially be helpful for patients who have lost their appetite because of cancer, chemotherapy, or infection with HIV. Few studies have looked at smoked marijuana to improve appetite, but Marinol, a synthetic drug that mimics one of the compounds in marijuana, has been approved by the Food and Drug Administration for treating weight loss in patients with HIV and relieving nausea and vomiting in cancer patients.

ARTHRITIS

Arthritis is an inflammatory condition that occurs when your immune system starts attacking healthy joints. There are three common types of arthritis; osteoarthritis, occurring most often, is the wear and tear of overused joints; rheumatoid arthritis occurs when the immune system strikes parts of the body resulting in inflammation and damage to the joints; and psoriatic arthritis, a condition marked by an inflammation of the skin and joints.

Symptoms

The inflammation of one or more joints, results in:

- Fatigue
- Joint pain
- Limited movement
- Swelling
- Muscle pain

Triggers

Although the cause of an arthritic flare up may be unclear, the following are common factors that may be the culprits.

- Certain foods
- Infection
- Fatigue
- Stress

Benefits

Cannabis-infused lotions increase circulation and eliminate swelling when rubbed into the affected area. Marijuana acts as a strong anti-inflammatory and it helps to reduce pain.

Conventional Medicine

NSAIDs (Nonsteroidal Anti-inflammatory Drugs) can be helpful in alleviating pain and inflammation in all types of arthritis, however they come with side effects, such as stomach bleeding and a risk of cardiovascular problems, such as heart attack and stroke. Acetaminophen (Tylenol) relieves arthritis pain as well, but it can induce the liver and kidney problems. Steroids may reduce the inflammation, but they can elevate the chance of infection, cataracts, and may weaken bones. DMARDs (Disease-modifying Anti-rheumatic Drugs) slow down joint damage, but not reverse damage, and that can lead to side effects, such as increased risk of serious infection.

Medical Marijuana

Evidence is present for the backing of medical marijuana in treating pain and inflammation associated with arthritis. Such an alternative is gaining accept-ance among the aging community to get relief from pain and for its anti-inflammatory properties. Marijuana smoked a few times a day is often as sufficient as NSAIDs or acetaminophen in treating arthritis, and without any fatalities. One of the main achievements of medical marijuana is euphoria or a state of well-being.

Canadian researcher Dr. Jason McDougall, a Professor of Pharmacology and Anesthesia at Dalhousie University in Halifax, has initiated research to determine if medical marijuana can help repair arthritic joints and relieve pain. In this case:

Katie M. of Madawaska, Maine, a sufferer of rheumatoid arthritis, began juicing raw cannabis after seeking the advice of a physician that specializes in dietary cannabis. She blended it into a smoothie and began to see results almost immediately. She was taken off her medications, prednisone and antibiotics, and after 11 months of regular cannabis juicing her condition is in remission.

See also **PAIN.**

ASTHMA

Asthma is a respiratory condition in which a person's airways—the tubes through which air travels to and from the lungs—become regularly inflamed. The inflammation causes the tubes to narrow, diminishing the amount of air that can be inhaled. People may suffer from asthma that is triggered by allergies, an occupational asthma, or asthma that is triggered by exercise.

Symptoms

Asthma sufferers exhibit symptoms, such as:

- Chest tightness
- Coughing
- Shortness of breath
- Wheezing

Triggers

Asthma attacks can be triggered by allergens, such as:

- Animal dander
- Chemicals
- Environmental pollution
- Smoke

Attacks can also be caused by:

- Adrenal disorders
- Anxiety
- Changes in temperature
- Exercise
- Stress

Benefits

Research has shown that medical marijuana can relieve the symptoms of asthma by either smoking or vaporizing medical cannabis without side effects. It relaxes and widens the airways allowing for more oxygen to enter them.

Conventional Medicine

Bronchodilators and corticosteroids are the medications most often prescribed. However, patients may be opposed to take these medications because of cost or possible side effects. Steroids are powerful drugs that can be risky when not taken correctly.

Corticosteroids may bring a risk of a number of side effects, such as glaucoma, fluid retention weight gain, high blood pressure, and psychological effects. Research has suggested that inhaled corticosteroids may suppress the rate of growth in children.

Medical Marijuana

An equally effective treatment for asthma is vaporizing and inhaling medical marijuana. It is a much safer, more natural, and equally effective treatment. If this is not a viable delivery base, cannabis edibles can be an alternative. Eating the marijuana edibles would have an effect on the whole body and be more of a preventive outcome. Vaporization as a delivery base is much faster and more direct and more advantageous for the asthma patient. The medicine goes directly to the lungs and the origin of the patient's problem, alleviating the symptoms right away.

To create a cannabis vaporizer:

- Empty the cannabis plant into the vaporizer
- Heat to the point short of combustion

Using the cannabis in this way releases the positive medical effects without any particles or poisonous fumes released, resulting in relaxing and pain reducing effects. It will allow the patient to calm themselves enough to not need an inhaler to breathe and decrease the dependency on

Medical marijuana dispensaries in major cities that have currently legalized marijuana can also direct you in the direction of good vaporizers. Very often they will sell the vaporizers with the medicinal marijuana upon request.

See also **ALLERGIES and INFLAMMATION.**

ATHEROSCLEROSIS

Atherosclerosis, or *arteriosclerosis,* is a buildup of fat deposits on the walls of your arteries. These deposits cause cartilage in the arteries to lose elasticity and the artery walls to become hard and thick. Atherosclerosis can lead to major health problems.

Symptoms

Atherosclerosis emerges slowly and usually doesn't give rise to signs or symptoms until it severely narrows or totally blocks an artery. Most people don't know they are suffering from the disease prior to a medical emergency, such as a heart attack or stroke.

Triggers

The hardening of the arteries caused by plaque buildup restricts the blood flow in the arteries, prohibiting your organs and tissues from obtaining the oxygenated blood they require to function. Common triggers of the hardening of the arteries are:

- Aging
- Diet
- Family history of heart disease

- High cholesterol levels
- Hypertension
- Lack of exercise
- Smoking

Benefits

According to researchers, it has been found that cannabinoids cause blood vessels to relax and widen. This results in lower blood pressure and improved circulation, lowering the risk of heart disease.

Conventional Medicine

Current treatments for atherosclerosis are mainly based on drugs that lower plasma cholesterol concentration and blood pressure and have significant adverse effects. Most often these medications, such as statins and fibrates, are prescribed to slow or halt the progression of atherosclerosis. These medications can present adverse side effects, such as headaches, trouble sleeping, abdominal cramping and diarrhea, and possible damage to the liver and digestive system.

Medical Marijuana

There is now notable evidence that demonstrates a therapeutic role of cannabinoids in a variety of heart conditions, including atherosclerosis. Since inflammation is a substantial feature of atherosclerosis, researchers have proposed that cannabinoids may be able to reverse the progression of this disease.

Steffens et al. (2005) were the first researchers to provide support for the assumption that relatively low oral doses of THC, initiated after manifestation of clinically detectable artery lesions, significantly inhibit atherosclerosis progression in mice. Their research cited that a 1 mg/kg daily dose of THC generated the most favorable response, which is much lower than the quantity of THC that results in psychoactive effects.

ATTENTION DEFICIT HYPERACITIVITY DISORDER (ADHD)

ADHD is a mental disorder in which the brain cannot overlook insignificant stimuli. It is a chronic disorder beginning in early childhood. The condition is also known as attention deficit disorder (ADD) however, ADD is a dated term for this condition. Adults are inclined to be diagnosed with attention deficit disorder as well. This condition is estimated to affect 3 to 5 percent of children and adults.

Symptoms

Individuals with attention deficit hyperactivity disorder experience trouble with self-regulation and self-motivation because they:

- Get distracted
- Lack organizational skills
- Lack the ability to prioritize
- Procrastinate

Triggers

A fundamental physiological irregularity of ADD/ADHD is the brain's deficiency of dopamine, a chemical neurotransmitter involved in cognitive processes like memory and attention.

Benefits

Ongoing research exhibits that certain strains of medical marijuana can allow the patient to concentrate on their task. Marijuana was used as a substitute for other medications (Ritalin or Methylphenidate). Chronic signs of ADHD are improved with the use of medical marijuana such as lack of attention. THC slows the ADHD brain's over-activity so patient can continue to be attentive to the job at hand.

Conventional Medicine

Medications like Adderall and Ritalin stimulate dopamine, therefore promoting concentration, but they occur with a countess number of unpleasant side effects and withdrawal symptoms.

Medical Marijuana

Dr. David Berman, who has studied the relationship between the cannabinoid system and ADHD, wrote "Cannabis appears to treat ADD and ADHD by increasing the availability of dopamine. This then has the same effect but is a different mechanism of action than stimulants like Ritalin (methylphenidate) and dexedrine amphetamine, which act by binding to the dopamine and interfering with the metabolic breakdown of dopamine."

"It seems to me if one is going to need to use drugs, one ought to consider a relatively safe drug, like marijuana," said Bernard Rimland, Ph.D. of the Autism Research Institute. Marijuana, the forbidden medicine, seems to be useful for some people with adult attention deficit disorder, impulse disorders, and bipolar disorder. Dr. Rimland continues saying, "Clearly, medical marijuana is not a drug to be administered lightly. But compare its side effects to the known effects of Risperdal, which include massive weight gain, a dramatically increased risk of diabetes, an elevated risk of deadly heart problems, as well as a host of other major and minor problems. Other psychotropic drugs are no safer, causing cause symptoms ranging from debilitating tardive dyskinesia to life-threatening malignant hyperthermia or sudden cardiac arrest. Of all drugs, the psychotropic drugs are amongst the least useful and most dangerous, and the benefit-vs-risk profile of medical marijuana seems fairly benign in comparison." He continues, "The reports we are seeing from parents indicate that medical marijuana often works when no other treatments, drug or non-drug, have helped."

AUTISM

Autism is a collection of disabilities, ASD (autism spectrum disorders), that impact brain development. The disorders can range in severity from mild to disabling. On the autism spectrum there are three different kinds of disorders; the most "classic" autism, autistic disorder; asperger syndrome; and pervasive developmental disorder, also referred to as "atypical autism." These disorders often materialize before a child reaches the age of 3 and lasts throughout their life.

Symptoms

Autism is characterized by:

- Communication difficulties
- Difficulty adjusting to changes in routine or surroundings
- Social interaction problems
- Repetitive and sometimes harmful behaviors
- Obsession with unusual objects

Triggers

There is no one factor that triggers ASD. However, autism tends to run in families and may be caused by a mix of genetics and environmental factors, such as advanced parental age and pregnancy problems. Autism experts claim that heavy metals may be the reason there has been such an increase in autism and other neurological disorders.

Benefits

Researchers have cited a link between increasing the natural marijuana-like chemicals in the brain and how it is effective in correcting behavioral issues related to autism.

Conventional Medicine

To treat autism symptoms, most physicians prescribe "off label" drugs, drugs that the FDA has approved for other disorders. Examples of these drugs are SSRIs (selective serotonin re-uptake inhibitors), such as fluoxetine which is prescribed for anxiety and depression disorders. To defuse debilitating repetition and harmful behaviors the "off label" drug naltrexone is prescribed. Naltrexone is commonly prescribed for alcohol and opioid addictions. These treatments do not do the job for everyone, and they may have side effects.

Medical Marijuana

Doctors are skeptical about endorsing cannabis in treating autism because of the scarcity of scientific data, but some favorable additional research exists. The endocannabinoid system consists simply of a group of receptors located in the brain and throughout the nervous system. This regulatory system, when out of balance, has an intimate relationship with many of the symptoms listed on the austim-spectrum. In addition, research shows links between autism disorders and impaired functioning of the endocannabinoid system. The chemical component of the cannabis plant, cannabidiol (CDB), is showing major promise towards helping to rebalance the body's endocannabinoid system and alleviate certain autism-related symptoms.

See also **CHAPTER 4, PAGE 29.**

BRAIN CANCER

See **CANCER.**

BREAST CANCER

See **CANCER.**

CANCER

Cancer is the name given to a variety of more than 100 diseases in which there is an uncontrollable division of abnormal cells resulting in a malignant growth or tumor in a part of the body.

Symptoms

Cancer can cause almost any sign or symptom depending on where the cancer is located, it's size, and if other organs or tissues are affected. The following are some of the more common signs or symptoms, however having any of these symptoms does not mean that you have cancer. If they persist for a long time or get worse than your should see your physician.

- Change in bladder function
- Change in bowel habits
- Fatigue
- Fever
- Indigestion
- Nagging cough or hoarseness
- New skin change
- Pain
- Skin changes
- Sores that do not heal
- Thickening or lump in the breast or other parts of the body
- Trouble swallowing
- Unexplained weight loss
- Unusual bleeding or discharge
- White spots on tongue or white patches in mouth

Triggers

Dr. Ryke Geerd Hamer, a German internist and creator of what is called "The New Medicine" in Europe, discovered that physical events combined with internal emotional reactions create what he called a "biological conflict shock" that will manifest itself as a visible physical transformation in the brain as well as measurable changes in physical-nervous parameters. From these central changes he saw the development of cancerous growths, ulcerations, necroses, and functional disturbances in specific organs of the body.

Some people feel that there can be no cure of cancer if the inner state, the soul, is not taken into account and cared for, but oncologists think this idea is absurd. But a 2001 survey of nearly 400 Canadian breast cancer patients by University of Toronto researchers found that 42 percent cited stress as one of the main causes of their disease, considerably more blamed either genetic or environmental causes.

> *Intense emotional stresses weaken the internal viscera,*
> *thus increasing the opportunity for pathologies*
> *of all types, including cancer.*

"There are few sources of stress in life greater than the words, "You have cancer." And we have known for decades that any kind of stress—especially chronic stress that's there day after day—has a suppressive effect on the immune system," wrote Dr. Paul McGhee. How we are treated during these moments when our reality literally inverts is telling and oncologists do use and abuse their power in such moments of our heightened vulnerability.

People are emotionally fragile when sick, and being told they have cancer or AIDS can completely shatter a person's emotional world. Goleman explains in his book *Emotional Intelligence* that this is due to the fact that normally "our mental well-being is based in part on the illusion of invulnerability." An understanding of vulnerability teaches us that a return to the vulnerable space is necessary and healthy. Vulnerability is the capacity or susceptibility to being hurt. It is not a weakness but a capacity to feel. For most people the feeling of being exposed to emotional hurt, or exposed to being taken advantage of, or abused relates to feelings of vulnerability.

Benefits

Relief from the side effects of cancer chemotherapy is a widely accepted medical use of marijuana in the United States. The American Cancer Society is one of dozens of national and international health organizations that have voiced support for further research on the medical use of cannabis in cancer chemotherapy treatments.

> *Cannabidiol (CBD) enhanced the susceptibility of cancer cells to adhere to, and be broken down by LAK cells.*
> —MARIA HAUSTEIN, PhD

Over 20 major studies have shown that cannabinoids actually fight cancer cells. In fact, it's been shown that cannabinoids arrest cancer growths of many different forms of cancer, including brain, melanoma and breast cancer. There's even growing evidence that cannabinoids cause direct anti-tumor activity. One literally has to be a fool not to consider utilizing medical marijuana in one's cancer protocol after reading the research as well as the experience of many people who have used it.

Conventional Medicine

The treatment a physician will recommend will depend on the type of cancer and the stage of the cancer. The treatment may include surgery, or radiation therapy, or chemotherapy, or all of them.

Both chemotherapy drugs and radiation therapy are powerful therapies that can cause side effects; immediate effects and long-term effects, ones that occur months or years after the cancer treatment.

Medical Marijuana

In 1991, 44 percent of oncologists surveyed said they had already recommended cannabis to their patients, and 56 percent said that marijuana should be legally prescribable. As early as 1975 the *New England Journal of Medicine* had reported that, "THC is an effective anti-emetic for patients receiving cancer chemotherapy." Since then, dozens of scientific studies recognized by the U.S. Food and Drug Administration and the National Cancer Institute have shown that the use of natural cannabis is a preferable remedy for adverse effects of the cancer-killing poisons employed in oncology.

According to Dr. Robert Ramer and Dr. Burkhard Hinz of the University of Rostock in Germany, medical marijuana can be an effective treatment for cancer. Their research was published in the *Journal of the National Cancer Institute Advance Access* on December 25th of 2007 in a paper entitled "Inhibition of Cancer Cell Invasion by Cannabinoids via Increased Expression of Tissue Inhibitor of Matrix Metalloproteinases."

Tetrahydrocannabinol (THC) and natural cannabinoids counteract cancer and chemical toxicity from drugs and environmental sources thus helping to preserve normal cells. Dr. Donald Abrams, a cancer specialist at San Francisco General Hospital says, "Every day I see people with nausea secondary to chemotherapy, depression, trouble sleeping, pain," he says. "I can recommend one drug [marijuana] for all those things, as opposed to writing five different prescriptions." Marijuana stems the nausea if one is inclined to go through chemo and radiation therapy. At the same time it treats their depression and just makes the patient feel better. On top of this it can actually treat cancer, reducing tumors and helps affect a complete cure. Medicine does not get any better than this except of course when one starts to combine medicinals (not pharmaceuticals).

> *The active ingredient in marijuana cuts tumor growth in common lung cancer in half and significantly reduces the ability of the cancer to spread.*
> —RESEARCH LABORATORIES, HARVARD UNIVERSITY

Marijuana cuts lung cancer tumor growth in half, a 2007 Harvard Medical School study shows. The active ingredient in marijuana cuts tumor growth in common lung cancer *in half* and significantly reduces the ability of the cancer to spread, say researchers at Harvard University who tested the chemical in both lab and mouse studies. Delta-tetrahydrocannabinol (THC) was found to inhibit EGF-induced growth and migration in epidermal growth factor receptor (EGFR) expressing non-small cell lung cancer cell lines. Lung cancers that over-express EGFR are usually highly aggressive and resistant to chemotherapy. THC that targets cannabinoid receptors CB1 and CB2 is similar in function to endocannabinoids, which are cannabinoids that are naturally produced in the body and activate these receptors.

"The beauty of this study is that we are showing that a substance of abuse, if used prudently, may offer a new road to therapy against lung cancer," said Anju Preet, PhD, a researcher in the Division of Experimental Medicine. Acting through cannabinoid receptors CB1 and CB2, endocannabinoids (as well as THC) are thought to play a role in variety of biological functions, including pain and anxiety control and inflammation.

Researchers reported in the August 15, 2004 issue of *Cancer Research*, the journal of the American Association for Cancer Research, that marijuana's constituents inhibited the spread of brain cancer in human tumor biopsies. In a related development, a research team from the University of South Florida further noted that THC can also selectively inhibit the activation and replication of gamma herpes viruses. The viruses, which can lie dormant for years within white blood cells before becoming active and spreading to other cells, are thought to increase one's chances of developing cancers, such as Kaposi's sarcoma, Burkitt's lymphoma, and Hodgkin's disease.

> *Cannabis extracts can shrink brain tumors by blocking*
> *the growth of blood vessels that nourish them.*
> —SCIENTIFIC AMERICAN, 2004

In 1998, a research team at Madrid's Complutense University discovered that THC can selectively induce programmed cell death in brain tumor cells without negatively impacting surrounding healthy cells. Then in 2000, they reported in the journal *Nature Medicine* that injections of synthetic THC eradicated malignant gliomas (brain tumors) in one-third of treated rats and prolonged life in another third by six weeks.

Led by Dr. Manuel Guzman, the Spanish team announced they had destroyed incurable brain cancer tumors in rats by injecting them with THC. They reported in the March 2002 issue of *Nature Medicine* that they injected the brains of 45 rats with cancer cells, producing tumors whose presence they confirmed through magnetic resonance imaging (MRI). On the 12th day they injected 15 of the rats with THC and 15 with Win-55,212-2 a synthetic compound similar to THC.

The Spanish team of researchers found that THC protected rats and extended their lives when they had cancer, also irrigated healthy rats' brains with large doses of THC for seven days to test for harmful biochemical or neurological effects. They found none. "Careful MRI analysis of all those tumor-free rats showed no sign of damage related to necrosis, edema, infection, or trauma. We also examined other potential side effects of cannabinoid administration. In both tumor-free and tumor-bearing rats, cannabinoid administration induced no substantial change in behavioral parameters, such as motor coordination or physical activity. Food and water intake as well as body weight gain were unaffected during and after cannabinoid delivery. Likewise, the general hematological profiles of cannabinoid-treated rats were normal. Thus, neither biochemical parameters nor markers of tissue damage changed substantially during the seven-day delivery period or for at least two months after cannabinoid treatment ended."

The cannabinoids inhibited the expression of several genes critical to angiogenesis known as the VEGF (vascular endothelial growth factor) pathway. Blockade of the VEGF pathway constitutes one of the most promising antitumoral approaches currently available, Guzman says. The cannabinoids work by increasing the potency of a fat molecule known as ceramide, the team posits. Increased ceramide activity, in turn, inhibits cells that would normally produce VEGF and encourage blood vessel growth.

The findings from Spain were first published in the April 2009 issue of *The Journal of Clinical Investigation*. The study showed that THC caused brain cancer cells to undergo a process called autophagy. This process causes cells to feed upon themselves, thereby destroying them, and not only did researchers witness this process, the specific route by which the autophagy process unfolds was isolated as well. Although this study involved injecting mice with live human brain cancer tumors, the study also involved two human patients who both had highly aggressive forms of brain cancer. When both the mice and the humans received THC, the tumors shrank in size.

Combining the two most common cannabinoid compounds in cannabis boosts the effectiveness of treatments to inhibit the growth of brain cancer cells and increase the number of those cells that die off. Researchers at the California Pacific Medical Center Research Institute (CPMCRI) combined the non-psychoactive cannabis compound, cannabidiol (CBD), with delta-9-tetrahyrdocannabinol (Δ9-THC), the primary psychoactive active ingredient in cannabis. They found that the combination boosts the inhibitory effects of Δ9-THC on glioblastoma, the most common and aggressive form of brain tumor, and the cancer that claimed the life of Senator Ted Kennedy last year.

Researchers at the University of Milan in Naples, Italy reported in the *Journal of Pharmacology and Experimental Therapeutics* that non-psychoactive compounds in marijuana inhibited the growth of glioma cells in a dose-dependent manner, and selectively targeted and killed malignant cells through apoptosis. "Non-psychoactive CBD [cannabidiol] produces a significant anti-tumor activity both in vitro and in vivo, thus suggesting a possible application of CBD as an antineoplastic agent."

The first experiment documenting pot's anti-tumor effects took place in 1974 at the Medical College of Virginia at the behest of the U.S. government. The results of that study, reported in an August 18, 1974 *Washington Post* newspaper feature, were that marijuana's psychoactive component, THC, "slowed the growth of lung cancers, breast cancers and a virus-induced leukemia in laboratory mice and prolonged their lives by as much as 36 percent." Funded by the National Institute of Health to find evidence that marijuana damages the immune system, these researchers from Virginia found instead that THC was astonishing in helping fight the war against cancer. The DEA quickly shut down the Virginia study and all further cannabis/tumor research.

"Antineoplastic Activity of Cannabinoids," an article in a 1975 *Journal of the National Cancer Institute* reports, "Lewis lung adenocarcinoma growth was retarded by the oral administration of tetrahydrocannabinol (THC) and cannabinol (CBN)"—two types of cannabinoids, a family of active components in marijuana. "Mice treated for 20 consecutive days with THC and CBN had reduced primary tumor size."

Ironically, the government's own National Toxicology Program study indicated that cannabis might actually help prevent cancer. In the mid-1990s, the U.S. federal government funded a two-year and two-million-dollar study by the National Toxicology Program under the review of the Federal Drug Administration, the National Cancer Institute, and other federal agencies. The study was designed to determine the cancer rate induced by injecting high doses of THC in the bodies of mice, then injecting them with cancerous cells. The study found that the mice injected with THC had a far lower incidence of cancer than did the control group.

The profound implication that cannabis use helps prevent and treat cancer was never officially released to the American public. The executive secretary of the Toxicology Program remarked many years ago, "I think it's terrible the way the government is handling this marijuana issue. There's no reason this shouldn't have been published." Compounds found in cannabis have been shown to kill numerous cancer types including: lung cancer, breast cancer, prostate cancer, leukemia, lymphoma, glioma, skin cancer, and pheochromocytoma, meaning many lives could have been saved if the government would have been fair with its own people.

> *Hemp oil can cheaply and effectively deliver
> a knockout blow to one's cancer.*

Hemp oil: Medical science is strongly in favor of THC-laden hemp oil as a primary cancer therapy, not just in a supportive role to control the side effects of chemotherapy. Hemp seed oil has long been recognized as one of the most versatile and beneficial substances known to man. Derived from hemp seeds (a member of the achene family of fruits) it has been regarded as a superfood due to its high essential fatty acid content and the unique ratio of omega-3 to omega-6 and gamma linolenic acid (GLA)—2:5:1. Hemp seed oil is known to contain up to 5 percent of pure GLA, a much higher concentration than any other plant, even higher than spirulina. For thousands of years, the hemp plant has been used in elixirs and medicinal teas because of its healing properties and now medical science is zeroing in on the properties of its active substances.

The essential oil derived from the crystals on the bud and upper leaves is not the same as hemp **seed oil**. There is very little nutritional benefit in the buds of the plant, but the THC carries the curative power in the cannabinoids and cannibidiols. Used as a tea, the leaves containing the THC crystals would be steeped and thus release medicine.

Rick Simpson tells us, "History calls hemp a panacea, which means cure-all. From my experience of seeing hemp oil used for various medical conditions, I too call hemp a cure-all. Hemp is useful in the treatment of practically any disease or condition; it promotes full-body healing. From our experience the oil is also very beneficial for most skin conditions; it can be mixed with skin creams or even suntan lotion. Wouldn't it be nice to go out in the sun and not have to worry about skin cancer? From my experience, the oil is effective in the treatment of all types of skin cancers, and the same holds true for internal cancers and other medical conditions."

> *If you treat leukemia with hemp oil it often produces very dramatic results quickly. Leukemia, from my experience with hemp oil, is one of the easiest internal cancers to cure. The first place the THC goes after entering the body is directly into the bloodstream. If cancer is present in the bloodstream, it won't be present for long.*
>
> —RICK SIMPSON, AUTHOR OF *PHOENIX TEARS*

Simpson continues, "Hemp oil seems to work on all types of cancer, and I am not aware of any type of cancer that it would not be effective for. Put simply, cancer is just mutating cells; THC kills mutating cells. When hemp oil is ingested as a cancer medication, the THC in the oil causes a buildup of a fat molecule called ceramide. When ceramide comes in contact with cancer cells it causes programmed cell death of the cancer cells while doing no harm to healthy cells. I have seen hemp oil relieve pain from bone cancer that morphine had no effect on. I have provided hemp oil to many people with chronic pain and some of the results have been amazing. It is not unusual to receive reports from people within days telling me that they are no longer in pain. Hemp oil has the ability to eliminate pain, but it also goes to work healing the problem that is causing the pain. Pharmaceuticals do nothing to heal the underlying cause of pain; they simply mask the pain. Realistically, there is no comparison between hemp oil and pharmaceuticals; most pain medications supplied by our medical system are dangerous, addictive, and deadly, while hemp oil presents no addiction or danger to the patient."

Marijuana increases our chances of beating cancer; it is that simple. Mainstream research leads us to the undeniable conclusion that marijuana is the premier cancer medicine humanity has been looking for and has finally found.

Contemporary oncologists are interested in it for its ability to mitigate the nasty side effects of chemo and radiation therapy. They never think of it as an important part of the actual treatment of cancer. The same could be said about sodium bicarbonate (baking soda).

Cannabis Science Inc., a pioneering U.S. biotech company developing pharmaceutical cannabis products, reported in early 2012 their success with self-medicated cannabis patients treating themselves for cancer. The case is graphic. One of the patient's physicians said it was the worst case of squamous cell carcinoma cancer he had ever seen.

Scientific trials have for decades documented the anti-cancer properties of cannabis and its constituents, yet it took the National Institute of Cancer, a component of the U.S. government's National Institutes of Health, awhile to finally acknowledge the herb's therapeutic utility for patients living with disease or suffering from the adverse side effects of cancer treatment.

See also **CHAPTER 4, PAGE 30.**

CARDIOVASCULAR DISEASE

See **METABOLIC SYNDROME and ATHEROSCLEROSIS.**

CHEMO-INDUCED NAUSEA

See **CANCER.**

CROHN'S DISEASE

See **INFLAMMATION.**

DEPRESSION

See **EMOTIONAL UPSET AND PAIN.**

DERMATITIS

See **INFLAMMATION.**

DIABETES

Diabetes is a metabolic disease in which the body is unable to manufacture any or an adequate amount of insulin, which results in high levels of glucose in the blood. There is nothing more needed in medicine today than a way of treating diabetes and metabolic syndrome because these syndromes lead directly to cancer, heart disease and stroke. Diabetes can affect the entire body.

Symptoms

The diabetes symptoms may vary depending on how much your blood sugar is elevated. Some of the symptoms include:

- Blurred vision
- Extreme hunger
- Extreme thirst
- Fatigue
- Frequent infections

- Frequent urination
- Irritability
- Sores, slow-healing
- Weight loss, unexplained

Triggers

The cause of diabetes isn't clear cut, but it may involve genetics and environmental factors. Diabetes and metabolic syndrome can be caused by toxic insults from heavy metals, radiation exposure, and chemicals running smack into major nutritional deficiencies. Diabetes is actually an extremely serious warning to civilization; it is an announcement that the rising tide of radiation, mercury, other deadly chemicals, and pharmaceutical drugs are poisoning humanity.

> *Populations are being simultaneously poisoned and starved by the food they eat.*

Diet, obesity, lack of exercise, and magnesium deficiency are also factors to be considered.

Benefits

The cost of not treating diabetes in a truly effective way is steep. Diabetes can contribute to, among other things, eye disorders and blindness, kidney failure, amputation, nerve damage, heart disease, and stroke. Diabetes makes pregnancy more difficult and can cause birth defects.

Conventional Medicine

"Conventional drug treatment for diabetes does not have a good track record. Prescription drugs have various side effects and are associated with severe health complications. Several researchers have revealed that long-term use of some common diabetes drugs can increase the risk of cancer and heart disease. An analysis of five-year data collected from an ongoing 10-year study, conducted by Takeda Pharmaceuticals, showed a link between the common anti-diabetes drug Actos and increased risk of bladder cancer," writes Dr. Marc Ott at Integrative Health of Orlando. Eighty percent of patients use two or more diabetes drugs every day.

The Food and Drug Administration (FDA) requires oral diabetes medicines to carry a warning regarding increased risk of heart attack. Medications for type-2 diabetes actually do more harm than good. In February 2008, researchers heading a large, government-funded trial made a sobering announcement. The Action to Control Cardiovascular Risk in Diabetes (ACCORD) study, designed to evaluate the effectiveness of various medication regimens, found that the most intensive drug regimens aimed at driving blood sugar way down resulted in a much higher cardiovascular death rate. Intensive blood-sugar-lowering treatment proved to be so harmful that the researchers halted the study 18 months early to prevent this aggressive drug use from killing even more people.

Avandia raises the risk of heart attacks and possibly deaths. Yet more than 6 million people worldwide have taken the drug to control blood sugar since it came on the market 12 years ago.

Medical science has known about the fatal complications of diabetes drugs since 1969 when results of a similar study called the University Group Diabetes Program were made public. That study also had to be stopped two years early because participants who were taking the drugs had a 250 to 300 percent higher death rate than those taking the placebo.

Dr. Julian Whitaker, director of the Whitaker Wellness Institute, says that, "The majority of patients with type-2 diabetes who come to the Whitaker Wellness Institute are taking at least one oral medication. We stop these drugs on sight. If they're on insulin and they're overweight, we stop the insulin as well. Giving insulin to heavy type-2 diabetics is a recipe for further weight gain and does more harm than good. As you might imagine, this is a new concept. Patients are conditioned to trust their doctors, who have convinced them of the absolute necessity of taking drugs to lower blood sugar. However, once they hear the truth about diabetes drugs, most of our patients opt to stop their medications and adopt a much healthier treatment approach targeted at lowering blood sugar and reducing risk of heart disease and other complications."

Most pain and anti-inflammatory medications are not safe; even the over-the-counter pain medications hold unforeseen dangers. Despite more than a decade's worth of research showing that taking too much acetaminophen can ruin the liver, the number of severe, unintentional poisonings from the drug is on the rise, a 2005 study reports. The drug, acetaminophen, is best known under the brand name Tylenol. Compounds containing Tylenol, include Excedrin, Midol Teen Formula, Theraflu, Alka-Seltzer Plus Cold Medicine, NyQuil Cold and Flu, and Paracetamol, as well as other over-the-counter drugs and many prescription narcotics, like Vicodin and Percocet.

Medical Marijuana and Magnesium

Diabetes is not the hopeless disease that most doctors would have us believe. There are safe treatments and lifestyle changes that will prevent diabetes from destroying your life. Cannabinoid medicine and magnesium chloride are a pair of medicinals that will positively impact diabetic treatment. Together they shame contemporary medicine's dangerous approach.

> *In studies THC essentially countered the effects of insulin resistance. These results support previous findings that smoking cannabis can reduce blood glucose in diabetics.*
> —GALLANT, ODEI-ADDO, FROST, AND LEVENDAL, *PHYTOMEDICINE*, 2009

Inflammation plays a key role in a set of disorders that include type-2 diabetes, obesity, and heart disease—collectively called the metabolic syndrome (or Syndrome X). Dr. Steve Shoelson, a Professor of Medicine at Harvard Medical School has focused squarely on inflammation. Epidemiologists have found that patients with type-2 diabetes and cardiovascular disease have slightly elevated levels of inflammatory markers in their bloodstream.

Magnesium. Magnesium deficiency is pro-inflammatory. Magnesium deficiency induces insulin resistance, hypertension, dyslipidemia, endothelial activation, and prothrombic changes in combination with the upregulation of markers of inflammation and oxidative stress. Though it is magnesium that modulates cellular events involved in inflammation, we can find another powerful and exceptionally safe medicine that can head inflammation off at the pass. When we understand the process of inflammation, and treat it with magnesium chloride, and other of my protocol items (cannabinoids), we can put an end to a large amount of suffering.

Inflammatory reactions in the body are a valuable predictor of impending heart attack. Magnesium deficiency causes and underpins chronic inflammatory buildups. Magnesium deficiencies feed the fires of inflammation and pain. Increases in extracellular magnesium concentration cause a decrease in the inflammatory response. Magnesium literally puts the chill on inflammation, especially when used transdermally.

Dr. Andrzej Mazur said, "Magnesium deficiency induces a systemic stress response by activation of neuro endocrinological pathways. Magnesium deficiency contributes to an exaggerated response to immune stress, and oxidative stress is the consequence of the inflammatory response." Magnesium improves and helps correct insulin sensitivity, which is the fundamental defect that characterizes pre-diabetes, metabolic syndrome, and even full-blown diabetes and heart disease. An intracellular enzyme called tyrosine kinase requires magnesium to allow insulin to exert its blood-sugar-lowering effects. In several studies, daily oral magnesium supplementation substantially improved insulin sensitivity by 10 percent and reduced blood sugar by 37 percent.

> *Let's not forget the sun. Researchers from Tuffs and Harvard are telling us that daily supplements of vitamin D boosts the function of the cells in the pancreas that produce insulin.*

Medical marijuana. Marijuana has strong anti-inflammatory effects. "This is why I believe that people who used marijuana a few decades ago are much less likely to develop any disease, such as Alzheimer's, that relies upon the slow development of brain inflammation," said Dr. Gary Wenk, a Professor of Psychology, Neuroscience, and Molecular Virology. The recent discovery of an endogenous cannabinoid system with specific receptors and ligands (compounds that activate receptors and trigger their characteristic responses) has increased our understanding of the actions of marijuana. Excessive inflammatory responses can emerge as a potential danger for organisms' health. Physiological balance between pro- and anti-inflammatory processes constitutes an important feature of responses against harmful events.

> *There is mounting evidence pointing to dysfunction of the endocannabinoid system having an important role in the development of type-2 diabetes and obesity. Insulin-induced glucose uptake increases with increasing THC concentration.*

Professor Mike Cawthorne, the late Director of Metabolic Research for the Clore Laboratory, and the pharmaceutical giant GlaxoSmithKline believe that plant-based medicines might be the way to approach the treatment of diabetes. The particular plant they are studying is marijuana. Cannabis is an excellent anti-inflammatory that lacks the side effects of steroids, the NSAIDS, and the COX-2 inhibitors like Vioxx. This anti-inflammatory action may help quell the arterial inflammation common in diabetes.

Cannabidiol arrested the onset of autoimmune diabetes in NOD (non-obese diabetic) mice in a 2007 study. Researchers at Hadassah University Hospital in Jerusalem in 2006 reported that injections of 5 mg per day of CBD (10 to 20 injections) significantly reduced the prevalence of diabetes in mice from an incidence of 86 percent in non-treated controls to an incidence of only 30 percent. In a separate experiment, investigators reported that control mice all developed diabetes at a median of 17 weeks (range 15 to 20 weeks), while a majority (60 percent) of CBD-treated mice remained diabetes-free at 26 weeks. Investigators also reported that CBD significantly lowered plasma levels of the pro-inflammatory cykotines (proteins), INF-gamma and TNF-alpha, and significantly reduced the severity of insulitis compared to non-treated controls.

CBD also occurs in almost all strains and is the second most interesting cannabinoid in regards to medical cannabis. Unlike THC, CBD lacks noticeable psychoactive effects. Nevertheless, CBD has valuable medical properties. CBD appears to work synergistically with THC, bolstering its medical effects while moderating its psycho-activity. It is also thought to improve wakefulness and to enhance THC's activity against pain. Taken by itself CBD has anti-inflammatory, anti-anxiety, anti-epileptic, sedative, and neuro-protective actions. It is also a potent anti-oxidant, protecting against chemical damage due to oxidation. Studies have suggested that CBD could protect against the development of diabetes, certain kinds of cancer, rheumatoid arthritis, brain and nerve damage due to stroke, alcoholism, nausea, inflammatory bowel disease, and Huntington's disease.

Researchers concluded that confirmation of the observed immunomodulatory effects of CBD "may lead to the clinical application of this agent in the prevention of type-1 diabetes" and possibly other autoimmune diseases. They note that many patients diagnosed with type-1 diabetes have sufficient residual cells that produce insulin at the time of diagnosis, and may be candidates for immunomodulation therapy. Immunomodulation is the adjustment of the immune response to a desired level, treating the disorder by inducing, enhancing, or suppressing an immune response.

Cannabidiol protects retinal neurons by preserving glutamine synthetase activity in diabetes. In current research on how to modulate cannabinoid receptors in the human body, Dr. Gregory I. Liou, a molecular biologist at the

Medical College of Georgia, has found that cannabidiol could prevent the overabundance of leaky eye blood vessels associated with diabetic retinopathy. As the leading cause of blindness in the United States, diabetic retinopathy is a major health concern for more than 16 million American adults.

Dr. Liou's work, published in the January issue of the *American Journal of Pathology* indicates that cannabidiol can interrupt the destructive points of action in diabetic animals. "What we believe cannabidiol does is go in here as an antioxidant to neutralize the toxic superoxides. Secondly, it inhibits the self-destructive system and allows the self-produced endogenous cannabinoids to stay there longer by inhibiting the enzyme that destroys them." Dr. Liou believes that cannabinoids act as a type of negotiator, trying to keep peace, harmony, and balance between a host of potentially volatile and dangerous factions of cells. "Cannabinoids are trying to ease the situation on both sides."

Cannabis is neuroprotective. It is believed that much of neuropathy comes from the inflammation of nerves caused by glycoproteins in the blood that deposit in peripheral tissues and trigger an immune response. Cannabis helps protect the nerve covering (myelin sheath) from inflammatory attack. Cannabis also lessens the pain of neuropathy by activating receptors in the body and brain. Some components of cannabis (perhaps cannibidiol) act as antispasmodic agents similar to the far more toxic anti-convulsants like Neurontin. This action of cannabis helps relieve diabetic muscle cramps and GI upset.

The *Journal of the American College of Cardiology* stated, "Collectively, our results strongly suggest that cannabidiol may have tremendous therapeutic potential in the treatment of diabetic cardiovascular and other complications."

See also **METABOLIC SYNDROME and NEUROPATHIC PAIN.**

EMOTIONAL DISTRESS

It is no secret that the most elementary neurological wiring in our brains is connected to the monitoring of basic biological system requirements—meaning, when our basic needs are met, our body's systems work much more efficiently. We have many legitimate needs for closeness, affection, appreciation, community, love, trust, understanding, and warmth that we often live without, and this is stressful in ways that are hard to calculate.

Symptoms

People respond in different ways to trauma or overwhelming situations. They may experience physical or emotional reactions, including:

- Anxiety
- Changes in eating patterns
- Changes in social behavior
- Compulsive/obsessive behavior
- Difficulty concentrating
- Difficulty managing anger

- Feeling sad or hopeless
- Forgetfulness
- Lack of energy
- Sleep disturbances/insomnia
- Unexplained physical symptoms
- Weight loss/gain

Triggers

Sometimes we are like Humpty Dumpy on a great wall, having fallen and broken to pieces, we still have to find some glue and put ourselves together. Pulling ourselves up by our own bootstraps is not the easiest thing to do but is often necessary not only for ourselves but for those around us who depend on us.

Emotions are energies that we feel. We feel our emotions and that is why we mostly identify our sense of self with emotions. Emotions are our way of feeling our thoughts. They reflect the quality of our thoughts, actions, and even our non-actions.

Many things can trigger these feelings. We could have just lost a job, a girlfriend or boyfriend or husband or wife. They say the worst is to lose a child; I can believe that and I hope I never have to face that. Many people around the world are losing everything at the hands of Nature, which is raging these days against us. Governments are getting meaner and are attacking their citizens and are even taking many of their lives. Most everyone at some time or another experiences the crushing weight of loss. I am speaking specifically of that moment when it all caves in and one feels crushed and washed away in a flood of tears.

Emotional distress or emotional burnout can be the result of situations that make you feel overwhelmed, such as:

- An accident
- An injury
- Loss or death of a loved one
- Natural disasters

- Relentless stress
- Surgery
- Trauma

A recent study from Australia prepared for the Climate Institute says loss of social cohesion in the wake of severe weather events related to climate change could be linked to increased rates of anxiety, depression, post-traumatic stress, and substance abuse. As many as one in five people reported emotional injury, stress, and despair in the wake of these events.

> *Deteriorating social mood is like a very slow-building, a very slow-moving hurricane: The longer it goes on, the stronger it gets.*
> —THE DAILY BELL, 2011

The study points to a breakdown of social cohesion caused by loss of work and associated stability, adding that the suicide rate in rural communities rose by 8 percent. The report also looks at mental health in the aftermath of major weather events. It shows that one in 10 primary school children reported symptoms of post-traumatic stress disorder in the wake of cyclone Larry in 2006.

Benefits

Research indicates the *balance of neurotransmiters affect everything* from sleeping, waking, love, stress, anger, optimism, pessimism, risk-taking behavior, and aggression to drug abuse, alcohol abuse, violence, anxiety, and appetite. It should be obvious that cannabinoids display their magic right here. Marijuana's neuromodulation effect helps us relax and calm down and this of course has a great effect on our health.

The most frequently reported sensations when treated with medical marijuana, include relaxation, drowsiness, emotional changes (usually positive), changes in how things are perceived and how time is experienced, and alteration of the actual thinking process itself. For medical or recreational-reasons, marijuana smokers usually like these feelings, at least once they get used to them.

> *Smoking marijuana offers small changes in consciousness, and this nature of change can work to smooth and even heal our hurt feelings.*

Although freedom from nausea and vomiting are two of the most noticed benefits of medical marijuana for cancer patients subjecting themselves to chemotherapy, many have reported a reduction in the severity of wasting away. They have also noticed a lessening in depression and other "side effects" brought on by the disease, including an increase in appetite. Bottom line is: Cannabinoid medicine has helped many cancer patients and people in general live better, happier, more comfortable lives.

In 2007, Katherine was diagnosed with rectal cancer and went through severe chemotherapy and radiation therapy treatments. In addition to being effective for nausea and pain associated with chemo and radiation therapy, using medical marijuana provided an emotional benefit for Katherine. "Going through cancer was a scary and lonely journey. I loved what pot did for my mind and thoughts. I could just unplug and daydream the time away rather than lie there scared and worried about what was happening to my body," she explains. "There is nothing like the mental and emotional relief of pot."

Conventional Medicine

The most common psychotropic drugs, such as Prozac, Paxil, and Celexa (SSRIs), affect the central nervous system and can alter emotions or moods. Although these mood-altering drugs work for some people, negative effects, including sleep, digestive, and sexual irregularities have been observed. There is also an increased risk of suicide.

Those suffering from chronic pain and severe emotional distress may have a high dose, high-risk opioid therapy prescribed. However, there is not enough evidence indicating that this treatment works, and research points to adverse outcomes, such as misuse, abuse, and even overdose, leading to death.

Medical Marijuana

There is nothing in the pharmaceutical world that offers the mental and emotional relief that marijuana does. Because of its nerve-calming and modulating effect, this book deeply explores the field of emotional medicine, treatments that touch not just on the body but also on the mind, our emotional and feeling selves.

The pharmaceutical industry will never come up with anything like marijuana though they do steal from the plant with extraction methods as well as synthetic creation. Marijuana is the safest most effective medicine there is for anxiety, stress, and emotional upset.

> *Cannabinoid medicine is the perfect medicine for stress and emotional upset. It is ideal for post-traumatic stress disorders.*

Certain naturalists and purists would rather us take nothing to deal with uncomfortable feelings or pain. But at some time or another everyone needs something strong because of overwhelming pain. Marijuana is perfect no matter the level of pain. Whether it is physical pain, emotional, and mental anguish or even spiritual pain, it can be attenuated with marijuana. We do not have to turn to toxic pharmaceutical drugs with serious side effects when we need pain relief.

Marijuana facilitates alternative states of mind that can be helpful in our search for peace within ourselves. In our struggles with self, with others, and with life itself, we often need soothing help and marijuana dishes this out with both hands. There is nothing wrong or dangerous in allowing cannabinoids to help us navigate the rapids of life. One cannot say this about any pharmaceutical.

> *Every person, at some time or other, undergoes painful life experiences. Pain and suffering are universal human constants. How we relate internally to our own personal suffering and the suffering of others sheds much light on the basic foundations of our personalities.*

There is no changing the fact that we are feeling beings. It is uncaring that hurts our beings, the lack of heart, and the steel coldness of the mind that is always seeking power, dominance, and control over others.

> *Life is a comedy for those who "think" and a tragedy for those who feel.*
>
> —HORACE WALPOLE

This tragedy of feelings can be mitigated with medical marijuana in much safer and effective ways than with any pharmaceutical drug. Cannabinoids can be used safely without short-circuiting our spiritual need to lift ourselves up by our own bootstraps, and in fact it can give us courage to face more calmly the distressing events and people that are threatening us.

GLAUCOMA

Glaucoma is a group of conditions that occur when the optic nerve becomes damaged. This condition leads to gradual vision loss and blindness. In most cases, glaucoma is marked by an increase of the intraocular pressure (referred to as the IOP) inside the eye itself. In some cases, however, while the optic nerve damage develops, the IOP remains normal. In such cases, medical marijuana treatment will not be effective. While glaucoma is more common in older adults, it can develop at any age. Glaucoma is the leading cause of blindness in the United States.

Symptoms

Usually there are few or no symptoms. If you have any of the following symptoms, it may be an indication that you may have glaucoma.

- Blurred or cloudy vision
- Double vision
- Nausea/vomiting accompanied by severe eye pain
- Pain, eye or head
- Seeing spots
- Sudden vision loss
- Tunnel vision
- "Watery eyes"

Triggers

The following are factors to help you determine the risk for developing the disease:

- Age (most common in older adults)
- Ancestry
- Diabetes, retinal blood vessel blockage
- Elevated eye pressure
- Eye injury
- Family history of glaucoma
- Family history of severe anemia
- Inflammation of the eye
- Steroid use
- Thin cornea

Benefits

Research supported by the National Eye Institute found that smoking marijuana lowered the intraocular pressure in glaucoma patients.

Conventional Medicine

The most common way to treat glaucoma and lower the intraocular pressure is with medicated eye drops; adrenergic agonists are a kind of drop that behaves like adrenaline. These eye drops may cause changes in pulse and heartbeat, dry mouth, stinging or itching, blurred vision, red eyes, or breathing problems.

Medical Marijuana

It has been demonstrated that medical marijuana lowers the eye pressure associated with glaucoma for 3 to 4 hours. The means of administering THC, the active ingredient in cannabis, include oral, sublingual, and eye drop instillation.

HEADACHES

Almost everyone has suffered a headache at one time or another, but many people suffer from various types of headaches on a frequent basis. While there are dozens of different types of headaches, these are the most common:

- A *migraine,* a severe to moderate headache, can be characterized by a pounding pain in the area of the head which can last for days.

- A *tension headache* or a *stress headache,* the most common in teens and adults, can cause mild to moderate pain

- *Cluster headaches* are reoccurring, severe headaches usually creating pain on one side of the head.

- A *sinus headache* is marked by a throbbing pain, with pressure around the eyes, forehead, and cheeks, which may be the result of pressure in your sinuses.

- *Hormone headaches* are a result of a change in hormone levels in women.

Symptoms

Migraines are particularly painful headaches often accompanied by nausea, vomiting and, sometimes, sensory disturbances called "auras." They can be accompanied by tingling in the arms and legs and increased sensitivity to light and sound. The most common type, the tension-type headache, feels like a tight band or vice is being pressed around the forehead. A day or two preceding a migraine you may experience:

- Constipation
- Food cravings
- Frequent yawning

- Increased thirst and urination
- Mood changes
- Neck stiffness

Triggers

Garden-variety headaches and their nastier cousins, migraines, can be triggered by sensory overload and stress, said Merle Diamond, a physician at the Diamond Headache Clinic in Chicago.

> *Migraines can be a totally disabling ailment that can render the sufferer incapable of performing even the most basic daily tasks.*

The greatest contributor to headaches is stress. Stress and anxiety can cause headaches directly, perhaps by disrupting brain chemical levels. Stress also leads to behaviors that make headaches more likely, such as poor sleep and skipped meals.

According to research presented at the American Headache Society's annual meeting in June, negative experiences in early childhood lead to more headaches in adulthood. Emotional abuse is the strongest trigger. Additional childhood stressors, such as parental divorce or drug-addicted family members, raised the risk even more, said Gretchen Tietjen, a neurologist at the University of Toledo College of Medicine and lead researcher of the study. Many of these changes take place in a part of the brain called the hypothalamic-pituitary-adrenal, or HPA, axis, Tietjen said. This axis regulates stress, memory, and emotions. Abnormal levels of stress hormones controlled by the HPA axis have been linked to migraines.

Benefits

Cannabis provides the headache and migraine sufferer instant relief and if taken at the onset of a headache, it can prevent a migraine. In addition, the frequency of migraine headaches is decreased with the use of medical marijuana.

> Marcy D., a former home health aide with four children and two granddaughters, never dreamed she'd be publicly touting the medical benefits of "pot." But marijuana, says the 48-year-old Ware resident, is the only thing that even begins to control the migraine headaches, which she describes as feeling like "hot, hot ice picks in the left side of my head," that plague her nine days a month.
>
> Duda has always had migraines. But they got much worse 10 years ago after two operations to remove life-threatening aneurysms, weak areas in the blood vessels in her brain. None of the standard drugs her doctors prescribe help much with her post-surgical symptoms, which include nausea, vomiting, loss of appetite, and pain on her left side "as if my body were cut in half." With marijuana, however, "I can at least leave the dark room," she says, "and it makes me eat a lot of food."

> Gabriel O. wrote:

> "I would like to give my opinion on marijuana. I have a history of migraines, the worst kind. When I have one I stay in a dark room from day to day, can't sleep or eat, I vomit, lose weight, and feel depressed. To top it off I was in a near-fatal accident. It took me 20 months to learn to do everything all over again. Ever since, I've had a bad back and can't work. I have spent days in the hospital with migraines. The medicine

they gave me was so strong I would sleep two or three days straight. They had me taking so many kinds of pain medicines I didn't know if I was coming or going. When I smoke marijuana it helps me sleep and eat, and I don't feel so much discomfort. I don't have a problem functioning like I did on the prescribed medicine."

Conventional Medicine

Federal health officials actually approved the wrinkle-smoothing injection Botox for chronic migraine headaches in October 2010, giving the drug maker Allergan clearance to begin marketing its drug to patients with a serious history of the condition. Botox works by blocking the connections between nerves and muscle, temporarily paralyzing the muscle. This toxin is made by the bacteria *Clostridium botulinum*. The bacteria themselves (and their spores) are harmless, but the toxin is considered one of the most lethal known poisons, one that has been a principle agent in biological warfare. It binds to nerve endings where they join muscles, leading to weakness or paralysis. Recovery from botulism occurs when the nerves grow new endings, which can take months, according to the FDA.

There are many common drugs that have been designed to treat headaches and migraines. Some of these pain relieving medications that may be prescribed depending upon the severity are aspirin or ibuprofen, triptans, ergots, or opioid medications, which are habit forming. These medications have troublesome side-effects that limit their long time use. Aspirin or ibuprofen if taken over long periods of time may result in ulcers and intestinal bleeding; the side effects of triptans may include nausea, dizziness, drowsiness, and muscle weakness; while ergots may worsen the nausea and vomiting related to the migraine.

Medical Marijuana and Magnesium

Marijuana is excellent at soothing the pain of headaches. Preventative medicinals like magnesium can halt frequent headaches, but painkillers like marijuana can be used to ease a headache already in progress.

Relaxation and biofeedback techniques that soothe the body have been shown to help migraine and chronic headache patients. In addition, in traditional Chinese medicine, acupuncture and acupressure has been shown to be effective in relieving migraine pain. As seen in Figure 1 on page 123, applying strong pressure to this point often provides instant relief from a headache.

Medical Marijuana. Throughout the years cannabis has been used for the treatment of headaches and migraines. Inhalation methods seem to provide

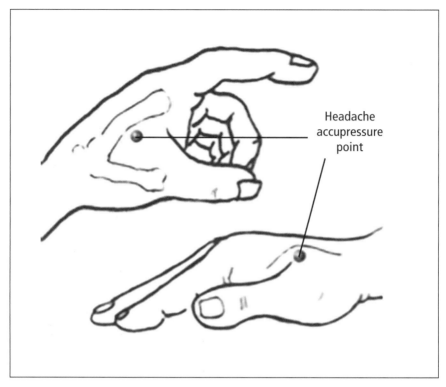

Headache
accupressure
point

Figure 1. Acupressure Point to Relieve Migraine Pain

the quickest relief and were more likely to stop migraine headaches and reduce their frequency, while edible cannabis takes longer to bring relief.

Prescription medications, such as antidepressants, tranquilizers, and pain medications, only treat the symptoms. Marijuana also treats the symptoms but in a much safer way then any pharmaceutical. Magnesium, on the other hand, treats the symptoms, while it simultaneously addresses the cause.

Magnesium. Many people needlessly suffer pain—including fibromyalgia, migraines, and muscle cramps—because they do not get enough magnesium," says Dr. Mildred Seelig, a leading magnesium researcher at the University of North Carolina. The problem is exacerbated when they load up on calcium, thinking it will help, when in fact, an overabundance of calcium flushes magnesium out of cells, compromising the effectiveness of **both** minerals.

Magnesium researcher Dr. Herbert Mansmann, founder of the Magnesium Research Lab, maintained that, "It's very likely that magnesium deficiency is a widespread cause of migraines." Studies show that many people don't even come close to getting the daily value of magnesium, which is 400 milligrams. "On a daily basis, 30 to 40 percent of American people take less than 75 percent of the daily value of magnesium," said Dr. Mansmann.

In the 90s cardiovascular biologist Dr. Burton M. Altura of the State University of New York Health Science Center at Brooklyn witnessed a therapeutic benefit of magnesium in acute symptoms, such as headache pain. Dr. Altura administered a solution containing one gram of magnesium sulfate intravenously to 40 patients who visited a headache clinic in the throes of moderate to severe pain. They treated migraine sufferers with cluster and chronic daily headaches. Within 15 minutes, 32 of the men and women—80 percent—experienced relief. Though the headaches may not have vanished completely, the pain lessened by at least 50 percent.

In 18 of these individuals, the pain relief lasted at least 24 hours. Blood tests before treatment confirmed that all but four in this latter group had ionized magnesium concentrations that were lower than the average in a related group of pain-free individuals. "All nine patients with cluster headaches had their acute headache aborted by magnesium therapy." Migraine sufferers who responded to the treatment experienced a complete alleviation of their current symptoms, including sensitivity to lights and sound. Subsequent studies of additional migraine patients have confirmed a common pattern, Altura says. "Those patients where ionized magnesium in the brain or blood is low will respond to intravenous magnesium very quickly and dramatically."

> My youngest son suffers with migraines. Typically nothing helps him except consistent adjustments from the chiropractor. The same night that I first tried this on my daughter for the constipation, my son had an awful migraine and was very sick from it. I took some of the magnesium oil and began rubbing his neck and the base of his skull with it. After a few minutes he said, "Ooh that feels good!" and fell asleep. When he woke up the headache was gone!!! Now, I'm convinced!!! I will never be without magnesium oil in my house! I am still stunned that this worked so quickly with my children.
>
> —Debbie G.

For a long list of testimonies on how magnesium helped migraine sufferers please visit the Magnesium Online Library site (see Resources, page 180). Mauskop et al. reported a deficiency in ionized magnesium in 45 percent of attacks of menstrual migraine, while only 15 percent of non-menstrually-related attacks had a deficiency. They also demonstrated that attacks associated with low ionized magnesium could be aborted by intravenous magnesium infusions. Facchinetti et al. demonstrated that menstrual migraine could be prevented by administration of oral magnesium during the last 15 days of the menstrual cycle. There is no shortage of evidence that magnesium is effective in reducing migraine frequency and pain:

- A 1992 study in Italy found that women with menstrual migraine who took magnesium at 360 mg/day beginning on day 15 of their menstrual cycle had decreased days of migraine and decreased total pain by the second month of the regimen.

- A 1996 study in Germany found that migraine sufferers taking 600 mg of magnesium daily for 12 weeks had 41.6 percent fewer attacks than they had suffered before the treatment. The beneficial effects were seen by the ninth week of treatment.

- A 2003 study in the United States (California) found the migraine-suffering children (ages 3 to 17) given magnesium at 9 mg/kg/day had a small but significant decrease in migraine frequency and severity relative to the group taking a placebo.

- Sodium bicarbonate also is recommended as another medicine that can cut a migraine to shreds or at least help the magnesium and cannabinoids work more effectively.

See also **PAIN.**

HIV/AIDS

See **CANCER.**

INFLAMMATION

Inflammation is the activation of the immune system in response to infection, irritation, or injury. Inflammation has different names when it appears in different parts of the body. Most allergy and asthma sufferers are familiar with rhinitis (inflammation of the nose), sinusitis (inflammation of the sinuses), and asthma (inflammation of the airways), but inflammation is also behind arthritis (inflammation of the joints), dermatitis (inflammation of the skin), and so on.

The inflammatory response can be acute or chronic. Acute inflammation typically lasts only a few days. This response usually promotes healing but, if uncontrolled, may become harmful.

Inflammation plays a key role in a set of disorders that include type-2 diabetes, obesity, and heart disease—collectively called the metabolic syndrome. Dr. Steve Shoelson, a Professor of Medicine at Harvard Medical School and Associate Director of Research and Section Head, Cellular and Molecular Physiology at the Joslin Diabetes Center, has focused squarely on inflammation. Epidemiologists have found that patients with type-2 diabetes and cardiovascular disease have slightly elevated levels of inflammatory markers in their bloodstream, raising the possibility that inflammation might be associated with the development of these diseases, and pro-inflammatory cytokines, such as TNF-α and IL-6, promote insulin resistance in experimental models.

> *Obesity without inflammation does not result*
> *in insulin resistance.*
> —DR. JEROLD OLEFSKY, PROFESSOR OF MEDICINE,
> UNIVERSITY OF CALIFORNIA

Inflammation itself has been well studied by immunologists: after an infection, a host of different types of immune cells are deployed to the infection site to control the infection. But Dr. Shoelson says that the situation is different in patients with metabolic diseases: the same markers of an immune response are present, but they persist chronically at low levels instead of following the dramatic rise and fall in an infection.

"Inflammation in blood vessels is one of the main drivers of atherosclerosis, and diabetes makes it much worse," said Dr. Jun-ichi Abe of the University of Rochester Medical Center. Dr. Abe said that in people without diabetes, fast blood flow triggers anti-inflammatory enzymes, endothelial nitric oxide synthase, and other factors, which block the ability of pro-inflammatory immune cells to hone in on and adhere to diseased portions of blood vessels.

A study done at New York University and published in March of 2008, found that pregnant women with periodontal (gum) disease have an increased risk of developing gestational diabetes mellitus than pregnant women with healthy gums. We see inflammation in diabetes with the inflammation of the gums spreading to the rest of the body through the blood vessels.

> *Inflammation plays a pivotal role in all stages of atherosclerosis,*
> *which is the progressive narrowing and hardening*
> *of the arteries over time.*

Symptoms

Inflammation is characterized by an influx of white blood cells, redness, heat, swelling, pain, and dysfunction of the organs involved. Symptoms of inflammation include the following signs at the site:

- Flu-like symptoms
- Loss of joint function
- Pain in the joints
- Redness
- Stiffness in the joints
- Swollen joints, may be warm to the touch

Triggers

There are many factors that trigger inflammation. They are found in both our internal and external environments and include:

- Certain pharmacological drugs
- Emotional stress
- Environmental toxins (heavy metals)
- Excessive levels of the hormone insulin (insulin resistance)
- Free-radical damage
- Obesity
- Overconsumption of hydrogenated oils
- Periodontal disease
- Radiation exposure
- Smoking
- Spirochetes, such as the Borrelia that causes Lyme disease
- Stress
- Viral, bacterial, fungal, and other pathogenic infections

Contemporary medicine does not recognize how subtle, constant and easily triggered inflammatory processes can be. "Eating induces an inflammatory state in everyone. Normally, inflammation occurs for three or four hours after eating but will then taper off. Though people can't avoid eating, Dr. Dandona says they can avoid what and how much they eat. He says, "If people eat McDonald's-type meals every three or four hours, and many do, they spend most of their time in a pro-inflammatory state."

Benefits

Studies have cited that marijuana is effective at decreasing the chronic inflammation associated with a variety of diseases. It can help patients curtail the pain associated with their inflammation-related condition, such as some cancers, rheumatoid arthritis, atherosclerosis, periodontitis, Crohn's disease, allergies (skin and rhinitis), and others.

When magnesium levels fall researchers note a profound increase of inflammatory cytokines present, along with increased levels of histamine. Magnesium deficiency causes and underpins chronic inflammatory build ups.

Conventional Medicine

NSAIDs, at prescription doses, reduce inflammation, however there are negative side effects associated with these drugs, such as stomach pain, headaches, dizziness, ringing in the ears, liver or kidney problems, onset of stomach ulcers, and high blood pressure.

Corticosteriods and prednisone may be prescribed as well to treat a variety of inflammatory disorders and diseases. These steroids may produce significant side effects and health complications. One may experience fluid retention, psychological effects, elevated blood pressure, glaucoma (an elevated pressure in the eyes), and weight gain.

Medical Marijuana and Magnesium

Inflammation plays a key role in a set of disorders. Magnesium and cannabinoid medicine are medicinals that will positively impact conditions and diseases associated with inflammation. Research has shown that these medicines treat these conditions without the various side effects and severe health complications associated with conventional drug treatments.

Medical marijuana. Cannabinoids have been found to reduce the inflammatory markers in chronic pancreatitis, to reduce skin inflammations when used topically, and to reduce inflammation in the bowel, proving useful in the treatment of Crohn's disease. Relatively low oral doses of THC, initiated after manifestation of clinically detectable artery lesions, significantly inhibit atherosclerosis progression in mice. Atherosclerosis is a chronic inflammatory disease that can lead to acute clinical events following plaque rupture and thrombosis. Current treatments for atherosclerosis are mainly based on drugs that lower plasma cholesterol concentration and blood pressure and have significant adverse effects.

The recent discovery of an endogenous cannabinoid system with specific receptors and ligands (a compound that activates a receptor and triggers its characteristic response) has vastly increased our understanding of the actions of an organism's health. The physiological balance between pro- and anti-inflammatory processes constitutes an important feature of responses against harmful events. Studies on the effects of marijuana smoking have evolved into the discovery and description of the endocannabinoid system. To date, this system is composed of two receptors, CB1 and CB2, and endogenous ligands including anandamide, 2-arachidonoyl glycerol, and others.

In an article in the January 5, 2006, issue of *Neuron,* the researchers reported experiments showing how the endocannabinoid anandamide (AEA) protects brain cells from inflammation. Such a role in the brain's immune system is distinct from cannabinoids' effects on neuronal signaling that produce the behavioral effects of marijuana.

Dr. Gregory T. Carter, Clinical Associate Professor of Rehabilitation Medicine, University of Washington School of Medicine says, "Marijuana has therapeutic properties that may be applicable to the treatment of neurological disorders; including anti-oxidative, neuroprotective, analgesic, and anti-inflammatory actions."

In test-tube experiments, researchers at the National Institutes of Health (NIH) in Bethesda, Maryland exposed rat nerve cells to a toxin that is typically released during strokes. Cannabidiol reduces the extent of damage researchers reported to the National Academy of Sciences. More effective than vitamins C or E, strong antioxidants, such as cannabidiol will neutralize free radicals and so might limit the damage and reduce the severity of ischemic strokes.

Magnesium. It is magnesium that modulates cellular events involved in inflammation. Inflammatory reactions in the body are a valuable predictor of impending heart attack. Dr. Robert Genko, editor of the *American Academy of Periodontal Journal,* claims that persons with gingival disease (which is an inflammatory disorder) are 27 times more likely to suffer a heart attack than are persons with healthy gums. An American Heart Association paper disclosed that 85 percent of heart attack victims had gum disease compared to 29 percent of healthy similar patients.

When magnesium levels fall researchers note a
profound increase of inflammatory cytokines present,
along with increased levels of histamine.

Magnesium deficiency causes and underpins chronic inflammatory buildups. This concept is intriguing because it suggests a fundamentally simpler way of warding off disease. Instead of conventional treatments for heart disease, Alzheimer's, and colon cancer, we apply natural inflammation-reducing remedies like cannabis and magnesium, which together would prevent or treat these deadly diseases. Inflammation and systemic stress are central attributes of many pathological conditions. In marijuana and magnesium we have potent medicinals that are effective across a wide range of pathologies because they both bring down inflammation.

Inflammation is the missing link to explain the role of magnesium in many pathological conditions. Magnesium decreases swelling, and, "is effective in the treatment of inflammatory skin diseases."

Magnesium deficiencies feed the fires of inflammation and pain. Epidemiologic studies have shown an inverse relationship between magnesium in the drinking water and cardiovascular mortality. This association between magnesium in drinking water and ischemic heart disease was reconfirmed in a major review of the literature done by epidemiologists at Johns Hopkins University. Since most heart disease is marked by various levels of inflammation, these studies were all highlighting the hidden relationship between inflammation and magnesium deficiency.

Increases in extracellular magnesium concentration cause a decrease in the inflammatory response, while reduction in the extracellular magnesium results in inflammation. Inflammation causes endothelial dysfunction and activated endothelium facilitates adhesion and migration of cancer cells. Magnesium literally puts the chill on inflammation, especially when used transdermally.

Heart disease begins with inflammatory chemicals that rage like a fever through your blood vessels. Cool the heat by getting the recommended daily minimum of magnesium, suggests Medical University of South Carolina researchers. They measured blood inflammation levels—using the C-reactive protein (CRP) test—in 3,800 men and women and found that those who got less than 50 percent of the RDA (310 to 420 mg) for magnesium were almost three times as likely to have dangerously high CRP levels as those who consumed enough. Being over age 40 and overweight and consuming less than 50 percent of the RDA more than doubled the risk of blood-vessel-damaging inflammation.

Dr. Andrzej Mazur, et al. have shown in experimentally induced magnesium deficiency in rats that after only a few days a clinical inflammatory syndrome develops and is characterized by leukocyte (white blood cell) and macrophage activation, release of inflammatory cytokines, and excessive production of free radicals. "Magnesium deficiency induces a systemic stress response by activation of neuroendocrinological pathways," writes Dr. Mazur. "Magnesium deficiency contributes to an exaggerated response to immune stress, and oxidative stress is the consequence of the inflammatory response," he continued.

See also **METABOLIC SYNDROME.**

INSOMNIA

See **SLEEP DISORDERS.**

LUNG CANCER

See **CANCER.**

METABOLIC SYNDROME

Long before diabetes develops, insulin resistance can be linked to a cluster of dysfunction changes known as metabolic syndrome. Inflammation plays a key role in these set of disorders that include type-2 diabetes, obesity, and heart disease—collectively called the metabolic syndrome. Dr. Steve Shoelson, a Professor of Medicine at Harvard Medical School and Associate Director of Research and Section Head, Cellular and Molecular Physiology at the Joslin Diabetes Center, has focused on the key role in metabolic syndrome, inflammation. Scientists have discovered that patients with type-2 diabetes and cardiovascular disease have elevated the levels of inflammatory markers in their bloodstream, which raises the possibility that inflammation might be associated with the development of these diseases and promote insulin resistance.

Inflammation has been shown to be linked to insulin resistance and to defective insulin signaling in non-obese diabetic (NOD) mice.

Symptoms

This syndrome often goes unrecognized because there are no obvious symptoms, there are however some classic signs:

- Blurred vision
- Excess abdominal weight
- Fatigue
- Frequent urination
- High blood pressure
- High blood sugar
- High blood triglycerides
- Low HDL "good" cholesterol

Triggers

This group of conditions—elevated blood pressure, high blood sugar, excess body fat around the waist, and abnormal cholesterol or triglyceride levels—may increase your risk of heart disease, diabetes, or a stroke.

Benefits

Marijuana, when used regularly, may lower the risk of metabolic syndrome. The *Psychological Medicine* cited a study including 1,800 adults who participated in the second Australian national survey on psychosis. The authors reported that those adults using cannabis in the 12 months of the study "were significantly less likely than non-users to have the metabolic syndrome." The authors also found in previous research a relationship between marijuana use and metabolic improvements among those not participating in this study.

Conventional Medicine

If medications are necessary to help reduce the risks of metabolic syndrome, drugs may be prescribed to lower your blood pressure, such as ACE inhibitors, receptor blockers, diuretics, or beta-blockers; to maintain adequate cholesterol levels drugs such as statins may be prescribed; or for glucose intolerance the drugs may include Glucophage, Actos, and Avandia. Each of these drugs present significantly dangerous side-effects and risks. For instance, common side effects for the ACE inhibitors are dizziness, headache, dangerously low blood pressure, diarrhea, drowsiness, and more. The most common side effect of statins is muscle pain and damage; although rare, liver damage may occur as well. Common side effects of Avandia are headache and nausea, but this drug has also been linked to heart attacks.

Medical Marijuana

Research presented in *The American Journal of Medicine*, found that adults who presently smoke marijuana are less likely by 50 percent to have metabolic syndrome in comparison to those who don't or have never smoked marijuana. These studies have shown a relationship between the use of marijuana and less weight around the waist, as well as lower levels of fasting insulin.

See also DIABETES and INFLAMMATION.

MIGRAINES

See HEADACHES.

NEUROPATHIC PAIN

Neuropathic pain, different from the common type of pain, is a complex pain that comes from a problem with one or more of the nerves. This chronic pain is usually related to tissue damage. The nerve fibers may be damaged for a number of reasons, including physical injury, poor circulation, and diabetes.

Symptoms

The symptoms associated with neuropathy depend on what types of nerves are damaged. Symptoms related with damage to the sensory nerves are:

- Numbness
- Pain
- Tingling
- Weakness in hands and feet

Damage to the nerves that control power and movement (motor nerves) may result in weakness in the feet and hands. When there is damage to the nerves that control body functions or the body systems (autonomic nerves) you may experience changes in heart rate, changes in blood pressure, and sweating.

Triggers

Americans for Safe Access tell us that, "Persistent and disabling pain can have numerous and sometimes multiple causes." Among them are:

- AIDS
- Arthritis and other rheumatic and degenerative hip joint and connective tissue disorders
- Cancer
- Defects or injuries to the back
- Multiple sclerosis
- Neck and spinal cord
- Severe burns
- Sickle cell anemia

Pain is not a primary condition or injury but rather a severe, frequently intolerable symptom that varies in frequency, duration, and severity according to the individual. The underlying condition determines the appropriate curative approach, but it does not determine the proper symptom management.

Benefits

Studies have shown cannabis is effective at significantly reducing neuropathic pain. Bioactive cannabinoids have an anti-inflammatory effect.

Conventional Medicine

For patients in pain, the goal is to function as fully as possible by reducing their pain as much as possible, while minimizing the often-debilitating side effects of the pain therapies. Most pain and anti-inflammatory medications are not safe; even the over-the-counter (OTC) pain medications hold unforeseen dangers.

The granddaddy of all anti-inflammatories is aspirin (acetylsalicylic acid or ASA), which can cause serious problems and death even when used appropriately. Despite more than a decade's worth of research showing that taking too much acetaminophen can ruin the liver, the number of severe, unintentional poisonings from the drug is on the rise, a study reports. The drug acetaminophen is best known under the brand name Tylenol. Compounds containing Tylenol include Excedrin, Midol Teen Formula, Theraflu, Alka-Seltzer Plus Cold Medicine, and NyQuil Cold and Flu, as well as other over-the-counter drugs and many prescription narcotics like Vicodin and Percocet, as well as morphine and OxyContin

Medical Marijuana and Magnesium

Chronic pain is a public health issue that is widespread across the aging populations of industrialized nations. Epidemiological statistics are alarming: in Europe, it is estimated that one in four adults has a chronic pain condition. In the U.S., it is estimated that at least 38 million adults suffer from chronic pain, and at least 12 million have used cannabis as a treatment. It is the character, severity, location, and duration of the pain that determines the range of appropriate therapies.

Medical marijuana. Dr. Gregory T. Carter, Clinical Associate Professor of Rehabilitation Medicine, University of Washington School of Medicine says, "Marijuana is a complex substance containing over 60 different forms of cannabinoids, the active ingredients. Cannabinoids are now known to have the capacity for neuromodulation via direct, receptor-based mechanisms at numerous levels within the nervous system. These have therapeutic properties that may be applicable to the treatment of neurological disorders, including anti-oxidative, neuroprotective, analgesic and anti-inflammatory actions, modulation of glial cells, immunomodulation, and tumor growth regulation. Intracellular changes and altered signaling of the neurons seems to be the principle effects of the cannabinoids in marijuana.

> *Cannabinoids reduced inflammation in the brain and prevented*
> *cognitive decline. Cannabinoids have also been shown*
> *to alleviate neuropathic pain.*
> —JOURNAL OF NEUROSCIENCE LETTERS, 2004

Marijuana can also be used to make topical creams to relieve neuropathic pain and tingling in hands and feet. Cannabis helps still diabetic "restless leg syndrome" (RLS), so the patient can sleep better: "It is recommended that patients use a vaporizer or smoke cannabis to aid in falling asleep."

Failure to adequately treat severe and/or chronic pain can have tragic consequences. Not infrequently, people in unrelieved pain want to die. Despair can also cause patients to discontinue potentially life-saving procedures, which themselves cause severe suffering. In such dire cases, anything that helps to alleviate the pain will prolong these patients' lives."

> *Nausea, appetite loss, pain, and anxiety . . . all can be mitigated by marijuana—for patients such as those with AIDS or undergoing chemotherapy who suffer simultaneously from severe pain, nausea, and appetite loss, cannabinoid drugs can offer broad spectrum relief not found in any other single medication.*
> —INSTITUTE OF MEDICINE, 1999

A 2009 review of controlled clinical studies using medical marijuana for pain relief, conducted over a 38-year period, found that "nearly all of the 33 published controlled clinical trials conducted in the United States have shown significant and measurable benefits in subjects receiving the treatment." The review's authors note that the more than 100 different cannabinoids in cannabis have the capacity for analgesia (painkilling) through neuromodulation in ascending and descending pain pathways, neuroprotection, and anti-inflammatory mechanisms. From 1975 to February 2011, there have been nearly 300 studies showing that cannabinoids and cannabis can help patients experiencing chronic pain. Some of the most encouraging clinical data on effects of cannabinoids on chronic pain are from studies of intractable cancer pain and hard-to-treat neuropathic pain.

> *Cannabinoids, such as THC, are capable of inhibiting nociception, i.e., pain transmission, at least in part, by interacting with spinal cannabinoid receptors.*
> —JENNELLE DURNETT RICHARDSON, ET AL, 1998

Cannabis is well recognized for its pain relieving effect. It is encouraging to be able to relieve one's pain without having to worry about major side effects. One study reveals that marijuana relieves pain that narcotics like morphine and OxyContin have hardly any effect on and could help ease suffering from illnesses, such as multiple sclerosis and diabetes. The research, from the

University of California at San Francisco, found smoked marijuana to be effective at relieving the extreme pain of a debilitating condition known as peripheral neuropathy.

Doubling up with magnesium and treating the legs and feet with magnesium oil transdermally not only reduces pain of peripheral neuropathy but works fundamentally to execute a cure by relaxing and opening up the blood vessels for better peripheral circulation and easing nerve inflammation.

> *Three puffs a day of cannabis helps people with chronic*
> *nerve pain and insomnia due to injury or surgery feel*
> *less pain and sleep better, a Canadian team has found.*

There are levels of pain that nothing seems to touch, but even this kind of pain can be reduced with cannabinoids. Cannabinoids are already being investigated for use with opioids to reduce pain and reliance on opioids. When magnesium is put into the mix, then not only do we reduce inflammation that is driving the pain, we also relax the entire nervous system, which is why I always recommend combining medical marijuana with magnesium chloride. Together these should markedly reduce the adverse effects and reliance on the dangerous opioids.

> *Cannabinoids reduce inflammation in the brain*
> *and prevent cognitive decline. Cannabinoids have*
> *also been shown to alleviate neuropathic pain.*
> —DR. AHMET DOGRUL ET AL, 2013

Scientists have found a chemical in cannabis that prevents some of the painful side effects that develop following cancer treatment with the drug Paclitaxel, particularly for victims of breast tumors.

Cannabis has also been found to be effective in relieving the pain of rheumatoid arthritis as cited in the September 13, 2008 issue of *Medical News Today*. In a double-blind trial, researchers randomised 31 patients to receive the cannabis-based medicine (CBM) and 27, the placebo. The CBM (brand name: Sativex) was in the form of an easy-to-use mouth spray that patients could administer themselves up to a maximum of six doses a day. The CBM consisted of a blend of whole plant extracts, standardized for content that delivered approximately equal amounts of two key therapeutic constituents from the cannabis plant: delta-9-tetrahydrocannabinol (THC) and cannabidiol (CBD). Mouse studies have shown that THC and CBD have anti-inflammatory effects, and that CBD blocked progression of RA and produced improvements in symptoms.

The researchers found that in comparison with the placebo, patients who had taken the CBM had statistically significant improvements in pain on movement, pain at rest, quality of sleep, inflammation (measured by a Disease Activity Score involving 28 joints [DAS 28]), and intensity of pain (measured by the Short-Form McGill Pain Questionnaire [SF-MPQ]).

Magnesium. *Transdermal Magnesium Therapy* offers an important breakthrough in medical treatment offering an excellent a form of magnesium supplementation that is just not possible with oral use alone. Transdermal medicine is ideal for pain management, as well as sports and pediatric medicine, and for diabetic neuropathy.

Traditional methods of administering medicine such as tablets or capsules get watered down and become much less effective due to stomach acids and digestive enzymes before they eventually get into the bloodstream. Bypassing the stomach and liver means a much greater percentage of the active ingredient goes straight into the bloodstream where it's needed, and in the case of neuropathy, medicinal properties are concentrated in the local tissues.

Drugs enter different layers of skin via intramuscular, subcutaneous, or transdermal delivery methods.

Imagine receiving your medical treatment right in the comfort of your own home, if you cannot get to the warm seawater.

Transdermal magnesium therapy is optimal for pain management, diabetic neuropathy, and inflammation. The combination of heat and magnesium chloride increases circulation and waste removal. The therapeutic effect of magnesium baths is to draw inflammation out of the muscles and joints. Magnesium chloride, when applied directly to the skin is transdermally absorbed and has an almost immediate effect on pain.

Dr. Linda Rapson, who specializes in treating chronic pain, believes that about 70 percent of her patients who complain of muscle pain, cramps, and fatigue are showing signs of magnesium deficiency. "Virtually all of them improve when I put them on magnesium," says Rapson, who runs a busy Toronto pain clinic. "It may sound too good to be true, but it's a fact." She's seen the mineral work in those with fibromyalgia, migraines, and constipation. "The scientific community should take a good hard look at this."

Lynne S., who was a patient of Dr. Rapson, has been using painkillers and steroids for years to try to ease the pain of her arthritis and fibromyalgia. Dr. Rapson started her on 675 units of magnesium a day. Within days, Lynne called Dr. Rapson to report a surprising change. "I went from being in constant pain almost throughout the day and night to having moments of pain. And for me that was a huge improvement," says Lynne, a former college English teacher. She dismisses suggestions that the change is a placebo effect. "I was not one day without pain, and now I don't have to take heavy pain medication," she reports.

When I received the following account from my research assistant Claudia French, who was an RN in an acute care psychiatric hospital, I realized that we should address the issue of magnesium and pain more directly.

Yesterday I witnessed one of the most amazing benefits of transdermal magnesium I have seen. I work with another RN who is afflicted with arthritis, especially in her hands, and frequent muscle cramping/spasms in her legs. She has been using magnesium but became lax. Before leaving for work yesterday I received a phone call from her begging me to please bring with me some magnesium oil, as her hands were so cramped up and painful that she could barely stand to continue working.

When I got there, her hands and fingers were very contorted in spasm. Her fingers were curled up and stiff and her legs were cramping badly. She reported they had been this way all day, and the pain was driving her to tears. She immediately slathered the magnesium oil all over her hands.

We were in report and she wanted it on her hands right away so the entire nursing staff watched, and within 5 minutes you could visibly see her fingers extend back to normal and the finger movement return. We could literally see the relaxation taking place. It was simply amazing. Within minutes her hands were completely relaxed and functional again and stayed that way the remainder of the evening. She also applied the magnesium to her legs and found relief.

About 30 minutes after applying the oil, she held up her hands for everyone to see and showed us the arthritic nodules on some fingers. She described how painful these always are to touch. But she poked and prodded them telling us how there was no pain now. She was able to continue working and doing the extensive writing that is a large part of our work without any further discomfort.

Pain relief and muscle relaxation for people with arthritis and muscle cramping is an important and significant benefit of magnesium oil. The rapid relief, visible to us all was really amazing! The following day she reported that she'd gotten the first restful night of sleep in many days. The pain was not waking her up.

A friend of mine called me a few years ago about tired, sore, and aching muscles from the strenuous athletic training to which he, a 58-year-old, was subjecting himself. He was putting in 20 hours of training per week for competition in his 32nd Ironman triathalon. He was using the magnesium oil but just a little bit of it. I told him to buy a gallon and dump whatever he had into his bath right away.

"I did the magnesium soak two days ago as you said with 4 ounces. The next morning I was better. Yesterday I did a 101-mile bike ride up a 6,200-foot mountain . . . was out in the heat (90 degrees) for $7\frac{1}{2}$ hours and then ran two miles when I got home. I am usually cramped up when I get home after a day like this and feeling pretty done in. But no cramps. Did another soak after the ride and run (I used more as my gallon arrived) and today I am not sore at all. I should be limping around. I did an easy $2\frac{1}{2}$-mile ocean swim and did another 6 ounces in the tub, then got a massage and my body is feeling good."

According to Dr. Cathy Wong, a German study found that mineral supplements increased intracellular magnesium levels by 11 percent and was associated with a reduction in pain symptoms in 76 out of 82 people with chronic low-back pain. London researchers provide strong evidence that magnesium sulphate produces pain relief in patients with PHN (postherpetic neuralgia), a neuropathic pain condition.

Magnesium deficiency is common in people with depression and chronic pain. Major depression is thought to be four times greater in people with chronic back pain than in the general population. It has been found that the rate of major depression increased in a linear fashion with greater pain severity. Thus magnesium, when applied transdermally, since good for both chronic back pain and depression separately, is the nutrition/medicine of choice for treating these sufferers.

OBESITY

See **METABOLIC SYNDROME.**

PAIN

See **NEUROPATHIC PAIN.**

PANCREATITIS

See **INFLAMMATION.**

PARKINSON'S DISEASE

Parkinson's disease (PD) is a disorder of the brain that leads to shaking (tremors) and difficulty with walking, movement, and coordination. Parkinson's disease most often develops after age 50. It is one of the most common nervous system disorders of the elderly. It sometimes occurs in younger adults and affects both men and women.

The National Parkinson Foundation reports that in the United States, 50,000 to 60,000 new cases of PD are diagnosed each year, adding to the one million people who currently have PD. In fact, it is estimated that four to six million people around the world suffer from the condition.

Symptoms

The signs and symptoms for Parkinson's disease may vary from person to person. The general symptoms or signs may include:

- Automatic movements (such as blinking) slow or stop
- Constipation
- Difficulty starting or continuing movement, such as starting to walk or getting up out of a chair
- Difficulty swallowing
- Drooling
- Finger-thumb rubbing (pill-rolling tremor) may be present
- Impaired balance and walking
- Lack of expression in the face (mask-like appearance)
- Loss of small or fine hand movements; writing may become small and difficult to read; eating becomes difficult
- May be worse when tired, excited, or stressed
- Movement problems
- Muscle aches and pains
- Over time, tremor can be seen in the head, lips, tongue, and feet
- Rigid or stiff muscles, often beginning in the legs

- Shaking, tremors
- Slowed movements
- Slowed, quieter speech and monotone voice
- Stooped position
- Tremors usually occur in the limbs at rest, or when the arm or leg is held out
- Tremors go away during movement

Other symptoms may include:

- Anxiety, stress, and tension
- Confusion
- Dementia
- Depression
- Fainting
- Hallucinations
- Memory loss

Triggers

There is no known cure for Parkinson's disease in contemporary medicine however, toxicities from heavy metals and chemicals run head on into nutritional deficiencies causing disease. Although specific causes are unknown, besides exposure to toxins and environmental triggers, scientists have cited certain genetic mutations that can play a role in Parkinson's.

Benefits

Clinical studies have suggested that cannabinoids possess antioxidant and anti-inflammatory properties that could benefit Parkinson's in motor symptoms, pain, sleep behavior disorder, and psychosis.

Conventional Medicine

Many of the medications used to control symptoms can cause severe side effects, including hallucinations, nausea, vomiting, diarrhea, and delirium. This is typical of pharmaceutical medicine, which only adds to the toxic burden and increases nutritional deficiencies.

Medical Marijuana, Magnesium, and Iodine

I am happy to say that Parkinson's and other neurological diseases *do* respond well to my Natural Allopathic protocol. There is sufficient evidence and testimony to suggest that people do not have to suffer with the worsening disorder that leads to total disability. Untreated, Parkinson's disease leads to a deterioration of all brain functions and an early miserable death.

Medical Marijuana. It has only recently been observed that some cannabinoids are potent antioxidants that can protect neurons from death even without cannabinoid receptor activation. It seems that cannabinoids can delay or even stop progressive degeneration of brain dopaminergic systems, a process for which there is presently no prevention. In combination with magnesium, cannabinoids represent, qualitatively, a new approach to the treatment of Parkinson's disease.

Dr. Evzin Ruzicka, an attending neurologist at Charles University in Prague in the Czech Republic said, "To our knowledge, this is the first study to assess the effect of cannabis on Parkinson's disease, and our findings suggest it may alleviate some symptoms," states Dr. Evin Rulcka. Thirty-nine patients (46 percent) reported that their Parkinson's disease symptoms in general were relieved after they started using cannabis. In terms of specific symptoms, 26 (31 percent) reported an improvement in tremor while at rest and 38 (45 percent) experienced a relief of bradykinesia. Relief of muscle rigidity was reported by 32 (38 percent), and 12 (14 percent) said they had an improvement in levodopa-induced dyskinesias. The respondents reported that the improvement in symptoms occurred an average of 1.7 months after they had started using cannabis. Patients who used it for at least three months were more likely to experience symptom relief than those with shorter experience, the investigators reported.

In a 2007 study published in *Nature*, researchers from the Stanford University School of Medicine reported that endocannabinoids, naturally occurring chemicals found in the brain that are similar to the active compounds in marijuana and hashish, helped trigger a dramatic improvement in mice with a condition similar to Parkinson's.

Dr. Robert Malenka, at the Nancy Friend Pritzker Professor in Psychiatry and Behavioral Sciences, and Dr. Anatol Kreitzer combined a drug used to treat Parkinson's disease (dopamine) with an experimental compound that can boost the level of endocannabinoids in the brain. When they used the combination in mice with a condition like Parkinson's, the mice went from being frozen in place to moving around freely in 15 minutes. "They were basically normal," Kreitzer said. "It turns out the receptors for cannabinoids are all over the brain, but they are not always activated by the naturally occurring endocannabinoids," said Malenka. The treatment used on the mice involves enhancing the activity of the chemicals where they occur naturally in the brain. "That is a really important difference, and it is why we think our manipulation of the chemicals is really different from smoking marijuana."

Magnesium. Evidence is mounting that low levels of magnesium contribute to the heavy metal deposition in the brain that precedes Parkinson's, multiple sclerosis and Alzheimer's. Many of the symptoms of Parkinson's disease can be overcome with high magnesium supplementation. In a trial with 30 epileptics, 450 mg of magnesium supplied daily successfully controlled seizures. Another study found that the lower the magnesium blood levels the more severe was the epilepsy. In most cases magnesium works best in combination with vitamin B6 and zinc.

Magnesium protects the cells from aluminum, mercury, lead, cadmium, beryllium, and nickel and is often used alone as a mineral therapy for successful chelation of metals, and is necessary in their chelation when stronger agents are used. Because of its nerve and muscle support, magnesium is helpful for nervousness, anxiety, insomnia, depression, and muscle cramps.

Magnesium comes out on top in the class of cerebral protective agents. Magnesium offers significant cerebral protection with a high preservation effect on neurological function following brain injury or in healing chronic impaired dysfunction like in Parkinson's and Alzheimer's diseases. It certainly helps in the case of stroke and that's why they are experimenting with injecting it the minute the ambulance shows up at the door.

Nerve cells use a brain chemical called dopamine to help control muscle movement. Parkinson's disease occurs when the nerve cells in the brain that make dopamine are slowly destroyed. Without dopamine, the nerve cells in that part of the brain cannot properly send messages. This leads to the loss of muscle function. The damage gets worse with time.

It has been shown that continuous low magnesium intake induces exclusive loss of dopaminergic neurons in rats. Magnesium exerts both preventive and ameliorating effects in an in vitro rat Parkinson disease model involving 1-methyl-4-phenylpyridinium (MPP+) toxicity in dopaminergic neurons. Magnesium protects dopaminergic neurons in the substantia nigra from degeneration. There is a significant and striking effect of magnesium for prevention of neurite and neuron pathology, and also amelioration of neurite pathology. Magnesium deficiency, over generations in rats, is tied to the pathogenesis of the Parkinsonism-dementia complex and amyotrophic lateral sclerosis.

The lack of dopaminergic neurons is reflected by a disturbed balance of the neural circuitry in the basal ganglia. Cannabinoids alleviate some parkinsonian symptoms by their remarkable receptor-mediated modulatory action in the basal ganglia output nuclei.

—J. SEVCIK, 2000

The following is a testimonial for a magnesium oil therapy:

"I have completed my first day of magnesium oil therapy on William who has had Parkinson's for over 20 years. I am hoping for a revival of functionality but not with high expectations because of the severity and duration of his symptoms. His condition before starting the magnesium oil was: he couldn't talk at all. Could not articulate what-so-ever! He was barely functional and did nothing voluntarily. No exercise and no attempt to stop drooling. The drooling was getting so bad and so constant that I was beginning to isolate him to his bedroom in his big recliner because the carpets are new here and the enzymes of the saliva stain permanently. And it appeared to be getting worse by the week. That's how he was. He also had started getting violent with me. If I pushed him too hard he would fly into a rage and hit me with whatever he could lay his hands on.

"I applied the magnesium oil twice yesterday and he woke this morning and washed his own face, cleaned his teeth, and put on his robe by himself—without being told to do these things. This is unheard of and hasn't happened for two years. What is more, he is not drooling. The drooling has been massive and absolutely uncontrollable for about a year. His swallowing reflex is simply going. He has had his nutritional drink, his coffee, his brain formula, fresh veggies, and scrambled eggs and hasn't drooled once. So, my hope is high. This is the best I've seen for a very long time.

"After only three days, interestingly, his speech has been much better overall. I am applying it faithfully three times a day all over him. I will just keep up the application and let time do the explaining. I am very encouraged by the improvement in speech. I honestly did not expect to see any results. His eyes are brighter, the concentration is longer and better, and the speech is much improved. By no means has he become a 'toastmaster,' but at least he can string two or three words together now and does not freeze up completely.

"Most recently he has been quite violent. For example he thrashed me over the head with a plastic ladle one day so quickly that he got in six or seven good thwacks before I could snatch it away from him. But since starting the magnesium oil, his demeanor has improved immensely. No more surly ugly looks, no more stubborn refusals to swallow or do something that I ask him to do. Great improvement and best of all he is now able to communicate so he can tell me what he wants and needs.

After 3+ weeks his speech is still much improved. It seems to be stable now. He couldn't give any lectures at Harvard, but he can make himself understood as to what he needs or wants. As I said prior to the magnesium treatment, he couldn't speak well enough to communicate anything."

—Nancy V.

Iodine. Long-term iodine deficiency appears to be linked to abnormalities in the dopaminergic system, including an increased number of dopamine receptors. It is argued that this raises susceptibility to dopamine oxidation, which in turn causes deficiencies of the antioxidant enzymes Cu/Zn superoxide dismutase, glutathione peroxidase, and catalase. Dopamine deficiency also leads to elevated cytotoxic glutamate levels.

> *Iodine is found in large quantities in the brain and the ciliary body of the eye. Lack of iodine may be involved in production of Parkinson's disease and glaucoma.*
> —DR. JAMES HOWENSTEIN, 2005

". . . The hypothesis that Parkinson's disease may be linked to soil and hence dietary iodine deficiency, associated with glaciation, is not new. In 1987, De Pedro-Cuesta concluded that Parkinsonism had the strongest links with 'Early life exposure to a geochemical imbalance, related to the last glaciation, associated to iodine washing out, present in soil, water, and diet.'" De Pedro-Cuesta reached this conclusion based on Parkinson's disease prevalence and mortality in selected age groups and similarities between current levodopa use and goiter distribution during the period 1920 to 1935.

As early as 1959, Warren also argued that multiple sclerosis was more common in regions that had suffered recent continental glaciations where it tends to develop most frequently in individuals who, as newborns, were fed milk from iodine-deficient cows. It has been hypothesized that a lack of iodine in fodder deprives cattle of thyroxine, a deficiency that in turn prevents the conversion of carotene to vitamin A. Milk lacking this vitamin also lacks the essential fatty acids because the latter, which form the main constituents of the myelin sheath, are oxidized rapidly in the absence of vitamin A.

A thyroid deficiency in rats has been linked to reduced myelin formation. Rat studies indicate that iodine deficiencies can cause reduced brain weight, limited myelin formation, retarded neuronal maturation, a lowering of the production of various enzymes, and slowing of the rates of protein and R.N.A. synthesis. Similar processes appear to occur in many neurological diseases.

> *In the brain, iodine concentrates in the substantia nigra, an area of the brain that has been associated with Parkinson's disease.*
> —DAVID BROWNSTEIN M.D.

POST-TRAUMATIC STRESS DISORDER (PTSD)

Post-traumatic stress disorder is an anxiety disorder that can develop after exposure to one or more traumatic events that threatened or caused great physical harm. It is a mental health condition that can take place after emotionally disturbing and distressing circumstances, such as war, an assault, or a disaster. It can become a debilitating condition and it affects your life and the people around you.

Symptoms

People who suffer from this disorder are often edgy, irritable, easily startled, and constantly on guard. They often involuntarily re-experience the traumatic event in the form of memories, nightmares, and flashbacks. They frequently appear to have a need to avoid feelings and thoughts reminiscent of the trauma. They sufferer from emotional numbing, which often causes demoralization and isolation.

> *Immobilization with fear elicits profound, potentially lethal, physiological changes (for example, dramatic slowing of heart rate, cessation of breathing, and dropping of blood pressure).*
> —DR. STEPHEN PORGES

They may also suffer from:

- Aggression
- Body aches
- Chest pain
- Detachment
- Dizziness
- Emotional problems
- Feelings of intense guilt
- Flashbacks
- Gastrointestinal complaints
- Headaches
- Irritability
- Losing interest
- Persistent daily thoughts
- Sleeping problems
- Trouble feeling affectionate

Triggers

Post-traumatic stress disorder results from an overwhelming assault on the mind and emotions involving a threat of death or serious injury or damage to one's physical integrity. PTSD affects between 10 and 30 percent of people exposed to traumatic experiences including combat, rape, an accident, terrorism, and natural disasters.

Dr. Dennis Charney, a psychiatrist and director of clinical neuroscience at the National Center at Yale University tells us that, "It does not matter if it was the incessant terror of combat, torture, or repeated abuse in childhood, or a one-time experience. All uncontrollable stress can have the same biological impact." The operative word here is uncontrollable. The key psychological aspect of PTSD is helplessness, the feeling that you are being threatened or your life is in danger and there is absolutely nothing you can do to avoid it.

> *A number of studies have found relationships between a helpless/hopeless attitude, psychological distress, and suppression of negative emotions with faster progression of breast cancer and other cancers.*
> —UNIVERSITY OF IOWA, 2007

Nothing does greater harm to a man or a woman than feeling that their life is in danger and there is nothing they can do about it. Scientists have discovered that great changes in brain chemistry occur when there is a danger and there is nothing we can do to escape it. The feeling of helplessness is a terror from which the brain has a very hard time recovering. Many beings have confronted combat, torture, repeated child abuse, rape, and violent assault; each of these provokes a common biological and neurological effect when the stressful event is perceived as uncontrollable, thus leaving us helpless. When we feel there is something we can do, we fare much better through traumatic experiences.

Benefits

Research suggests that people with PTSD often use cannabis to help cope with their condition, citing that the use:

- Improves quality of life
- Reduces pain
- Reduces stress
- Sleeping aid, acts as

Some veterans and sexual assault victims use marijuana to relieve PTSD symptoms. The following are testimonies citing how medical marijuana has made a difference:

Paul C. suffers from PTSD and his wife, Victoria, says marijuana has made a big difference. "He's a different person. He's a better person.

He's more open. He's more communicative," she says. "At one point, we almost got a divorce, and I can honestly say that I think medical cannabis saved our marriage and our family."

Veterans:

One veteran who uses marijuana frequently says it helps him concentrate on creative matters. He says he's not sure how much it actually helps his PTSD. He feels that is a matter of effectively addressing the issues causing the PTSD; in other words, marijuana or anything else is no replacement for the hard work necessary in recognizing why something is troubling an individual. But, still, he feels marijuana is a responsible, positive factor in his life.

Another veteran who has used marijuana off and on for decades sees its usage as positive for balancing out life's frustrations and difficulties. He laughs and says his wife will testify to how nice it makes him. But, he adds, it can be abused. "Too much of the stuff and it will make you stupid," he said. "What's important is to 'understand thyself,' then come to an understanding what effects, good and bad, marijuana has for you."

Michael M., a 46-year-old vet, went to Vietnam right after his 18th birthday. The first night when his company lost their first men he recalls, "I sat in the dark by myself wondering what the hell had happened. I asked myself where these souls went, and was there a heaven for men who died the way they did. As I stared into the darkness I heard a voice behind me say 'Man, you shouldn't be out here by yourself thinking about this shit or you'll go nuts.' I couldn't look him in the face and didn't even look up for fear that he would see the tears in my eyes. He told me I needed to get drunk to forget it and go on, or I would die there. I told him I didn't drink, and he said he would be right back. When he returned he had a big joint and asked if I had tried pot before. I told him that I had a couple of times. He said this was about 100 times stronger than anything in the States and I should only smoke a little. Then he left.

That night alone in the dark, I smoked the whole thing, and I've never regretted it. He had given me my mental survival tool. It did not make me forget, just allowed me to digest the pain and fear peacefully and respectfully with dignity. Pot was no longer just a party high for me but a survival tool. I used it to cope with everyday things that others seemed to do on their own, going out, seeing friends, working. I was just another bombed-out crazy vet, useless, suicidal, and violent. I've had a lot of women in my life who liked me but could not stand the mood swings, the striking out and fighting, and the depression. After a while they all would learn the same thing: that when I had pot, I was nicer and more romantic and didn't get into fights. So they made sure I had pot even if they had to buy it for me."

Sexual Assault:

> *Women suffering from post-traumatic stress as a result of sexual assaults are being prescribed psychiatric medicines, even though there's plenty of anecdotal evidence that medical cannabis is a better solution.*

D., a 26-year-old woman from the north of Israel, says she began to suffer from nightmares about seven years ago after her partner raped her. After undergoing various forms of therapy, she thought she had largely put the trauma behind her. Then, two years ago, she chanced to see the rapist not far from her home. The nightmares came swarming back.

"I fell into a depression that went on until not long ago, during which I hardly slept or ate," she says in a quiet voice. "My whole life turned upside down. I left my job. Everything came to a stop. I went back to taking antidepressants and tranquilizers—Cipralex, Lustral and Prozac, and sleeping pills that made me addicted. It was a nightmare. There was no way I could get through the day without those pills. Then I discovered cannabis."

For D., marijuana is not a drug but a medicine. "When I smoked, I didn't need medicines," she says. "It didn't make my life good and beautiful, but it did make it bearable." She now shuns the array of medicines and sleeping pills she took because of the side effects. "I refuse to take antidepressants because of the huge amount of weight I put on, and which I was able to shed only after I stopped taking them," she adds. "They also gave me constant stomachaches, made me nauseous and itchy, and caused dry skin and headaches. That's what life with medicinal drugs is like. So, yes, I'm not depressed. I don't want to die, but I also don't want to live. I'm not me, I don't feel anything, I'm some kind of robot—not happy, not sad, not anything. I am a straight line. It's not a life."

Conventional Medicine

The conventional treatment in hospitals for post-traumatic stress disorder (PTSD) fuses psychology—in the form of cognitive therapy techniques—with psychiatric medicines, including anti-anxiety medications, sleeping pills, and antidepressants. But in recent years, researchers around the world have begun to probe more natural treatments, notably medical marijuana.

These medications are among the most common ways to treat post-traumatic stress disorder and the insomnia, anger, nightmares, and anxiety that often come with it. They don't really help much and actually make the situation worse because of the many serious side effects. A study in the *Journal of the American Medical Association* suggested Risperdal, a widely prescribed antipsychotic, is no more effective in treating PTSD than placebos.

Medical Marijuana

New Mexico has passed legislation authorizing medical cannabis for soldiers who returned from a tour of duty in Iraq or Afghanistan suffering from PTSD. One-fourth of New Mexico's 1,600 medical marijuana patients are PTSD sufferers. About 6.8 percent of Americans will develop PTSD at some point in their lives. A drug that could help prevent it would be remarkably helpful.

Dozens of soldiers who suffer from PTSD as a result of their army service in Israel were, and continue to be, treated with medical cannabis with the authorization and support of the Health Ministry and the Ministry of Defense. Dr. Yehuda Baruch, the chair of the Health Ministry's advisory board for medical cannabis in Israel, recognizes the effectiveness of marijuana for PTSD sufferers.

> *Over the last 30 years increasing evidence has been found for the existence of complex links between the immune system, the central nervous system and the endocrine system on the one hand, and psychological phenomena on the other.*
>
> —Van Gent, et al.

Most doctors are still loath to connect body chemistry with emotions, but neurobiologists know that neural and other biologically measurable changes accompany PTSD. There are times when emotions just careen out of control, and we need to medicate them.

The hypothesis that marijuana is effective in treating PTSD was confirmed in experiments, including a famous experiment carried out by Dr. George Fraser, a Canadian psychiatrist with abundant experience in treating soldiers with PTSD. He observed significant improvement in 70 percent of the soldiers who took part in that research, particularly in regard to their sleep. And why do we examine sleep in particular? Because sleep is essential, and one of the most debilitating phenomena common to PTSD sufferers is their inability to sleep: they are afflicted by nightmares and are afraid to fall asleep.

Professor Rafael Meshulam, an Israel Prize laureate for chemistry and one of that country's leading experts in medical cannabis, and Dr. Irit Akirav, from the Department of Psychology at the University of Haifa, have shown, in separate research, some of the marked advantages of cannabinoid treatment. "Cannabis is a medicine in every respect," Prof. Meshulam says. He does not understand the reluctance of many psychiatrists to make use of the substance on the grounds that it is dangerous and addictive. "The great majority of them are simply uninformed, period," he believes. Dr. Ilya Reznik, an expert on the subject and medical director of the Israel Institute for Diagnostic Neuropsychiatry thinks, "On this issue, the medical establishment is divided into two: 95 percent are neutral-to-negative about cannabis, and the rest are neutral-to-positive. No more. Why? It's conservatism. They were always taught that cannabis is bad, that cannabis is a drug, and the moment they hear the word 'cannabis' they see handcuffs looming on the horizon. So they run from it."

In a study published in the journal *Neuropsychopharmacology*, Israeli scientists showed that injections of so-called "cannabinoid" compounds extracted from marijuana blocked development of PTSD-like symptoms in rodents that had been subjected to extreme stress. Researchers exposed rats to severe, Navy Seal-level stress, including restraint, forced swims, and anesthetization. PTSD symptoms disappeared in the rats that were given cannabis two or 24 hours after experiencing trauma. "This indicates that the marijuana prevented the development of post-trauma symptoms in the rat model," said Israeli physician Irit Akirav, who published his study in the *Journal of Neuroscience*.

QUADRIPLEGIA

Quadriplegia, also known as tetraplegia, is a paralysis caused by illness or injury to a human that results in the partial or total loss of use of all their limbs and torso. The loss is commonly a sensory and motor loss resulting in a loss of sensation and control.

Symptoms

Quadriplegia is a medical condition that is often accompanied by severe symptoms and signs, including:

- Bowel incontinence
- Breathing difficulties
- Loss of sensation in arms and legs
- Loss of ability to intentionally move arms and legs
- Impotence
- Incontinence of bladder and bowels
- Painful muscle spasms
- Paralysis of arms
- Paralysis of legs
- Pressure sores
- Urinary incontinence

Triggers

The most common cause of these spinal injuries is traumatic causes, such as accidental injuries (car accidents or sport injuries), or work-related injuries. There are also a number of medical sources, for example causes related to tumors, a parasite disease, spinal cord infarction or myelomalacia, aortic aneurysms, and others.

Benefits

Research has indicated that medical marijuana can be most effective in spinal cord injuries and its related side effect, for example it can:

- Open up bronchial tubes
- Reduces pain
- Reduces spasms

Conventional Medicine

The damage resulting from the spinal cord injury spreads to cells outside the injured area causing nerve cells to die. Very often, corticosteroid, methylprednisolone (Medrol) is prescribed to prevent the spread of the damage. Methylprednisolone can cause dangerous side effects, such as:

- Bloody stools
- High blood pressure
- Increased urination
- Nausea
- Pancreatitis
- Shortness of breath
- Vision problems
- Vomiting
- Weight gain

This is not a complete list and there are other less serious side effects.

Medical Marijuana

Studies have shown that cannabis has the capacity to offer comfort for a diversity of symptoms related to spinal cord injuries, such as depression, pain, and insomnia. Cannabinoids can treat pain, reduces spasticity, and improves motor control. THC also has a medical benefit in its potential to provide an improvement in bladder and bowel control, pain, and insomnia.

See also **SPINAL CORD INJURY/DISEASE.**

RADIATION EXPOSURE

A number of types of radiation, labeled ionizing radiation, can be harmful. Approximately half of the radiation we are subjected to comes from nature; the atmosphere and the soil. The other half we attain from sources such as, medical tests, treatments, and nuclear power plants. Radiation therapy is the medical use of ionizing radiation as part of cancer treatment to control malignant cells; targeted energy used to wipe out cancer cells or tumors and to ease certain symptoms associated with cancer.

Symptoms

Exposure to large doses of ionizing radiation may result in radiation sickness or poisoning. Some of the symptoms you may experience from radiation therapy are:

- Anemia
- Bleeding
- Dehydration
- Diarrhea
- Fatigue
- Hair loss
- Loss of appetite
- Mouth ulcers
- Nausea
- Recurrent infections
- Red itchy skin
- Sloughing of skin
- Vomiting
- Weakness
- Weight loss

The severity of the symptoms largely depends on the type and strength of the radiation, the amount, and the length of time exposed.

Triggers

Every toxic exposure increases people's vulnerability to radiation. Toxic accumulation, whether from heavy metals, chemicals, pesticides, food additives or preservatives will each take their toll, weakening our resistance to it or our ability to clear radioactive particles from our bodies. Though the situation in northern Japan is dire, we have a situation of intense exposure with many forms of toxins surrounding us and our children that are not going to go away for the duration of our and their lives.

Benefits

Radiation sickness or poisoning is the result of high-energy radiation destroying or damaging particular cells in the body during, for example, at the site of a nuclear industrial accident. However, low-dose radiation, for example from X-ray exams, usually does not result in radiation sickness. Medical marijuana will reduce some of the symptoms.

Conventional Medicine

Contemporary medicine is committing a form of mass murder by not responding to the need to reduce people's exposure to chemicals, radiation and heavy metals; instead they choose to increase that exposure. Hopefully, new paradigms of medicine and dentistry will embrace a reduction of exposure to poisons as its most fundamental principle.

Today more than ever before we need a new paradigm for allopathic medicine! Since we cannot get rid of the field of contemporary medicine, it needs to be reformed from the inside out, and the only way to do that is to get into the underlying structure of its principles and practices and change them on a foundational level.

To be honest we know that this is as impossible as bringing Fukushima under control. We need doctors, especially pediatric oncologists, to understand that in an age of toxicity where patients are being heavily exposed to heavy metals, chemicals, and radioactive particles, the last thing they need is exposure to more of the same via medical treatments and diagnostic procedures.

Not only can radioactive materials escape into the air and breathed into the lungs at the time of a radiological emergency, but it can contaminate the food we eat and the water we drink. There are some medical treatments available for controlling or removing internal contamination. The treatments available to the medical professional are Potassium Iodide (KI), Prussian Blue, and DTPA (Diethylenetriamine pentaacetate). However, some of these medication come with side effects and health risks, such as constipation and upset stomach (Prussian Blue), vomiting , diarrhea, chills, fever, and muscle cramps, chest pain, headache, and light headedness (DPTA).

Medical Marijuana

Cannabis is also an excellent treatment for radiation sickness and exposure. Some of the benefits of treating radiation sickness using medical marijuana are:

- Increased appetite
- Reduced nausea
- Reduced vomiting
- Sleeping aid
- Weight gain

Scientific trials have for decades documented the anti-cancer properties of cannabis and its constituents. However, not until recently did the National Institute of Cancer, a component of the U.S. government's National Institutes of Health, finally acknowledge the herb's therapeutic utility for patients living with disease or suffering from the adverse side effects of cancer treatment.

Rick Simpson (who has already been mentioned several times earlier in this book), the man in Canada who has helped many cancer sufferers with THC-laden hemp oil, has a lot to say to people as we go into our increasingly irradiated future. "If used properly high quality hemp oil can provide a solution that will be of great help to mankind in alleviating the effects of increasing radiation. With all the radiation that is now entering our atmosphere, it is basically urgent that we now all start ingesting this oil as soon as possible to undo the damage this radiation will cause. Through my experience with the use of this oil, I have found that there is nothing more effective or more harmless that can reduce the damage caused by radiation.

I have seen patients that were suffering from cancer who were badly damaged by the effects of radiation treatments who were able to completely eliminate the damage in a short time. Some who have come to me who had radiation treatments were burned so badly by its effects that their skin looked like red leather. After ingesting the oil treatment their skin went back to its normal healthy state and the radiation burns disappeared completely. If the oil can do this for someone that was badly damaged by such so-called medical treatments, would its use not be effective to combat the effects of the radiation, now emanating from Japan? Now with the menace that all this escaping radiation presents, we would have to be insane to turn our backs on the use of hemp extracts to help us all deal with this situation."

National Institute of Health (NIH) in Bethesda, Maryland exposed rat nerve cells to a toxin that is typically released during strokes. Cannabidiol reduces the extent of damage reported the National Academy of Sciences. More effective than vitamins C or E, strong antioxidants such as cannabidiol will neutralize free radicals and so might limit the damage and reduce the severity of radiation.

RESTLESS LEG SYNDROME (RLS)

See **SLEEP DISORDERS.**

SEIZURES

The cells of our brain intensively exchange information among each other using electrical and chemical signals. This is a prerequisite for the brain to work properly. However, if the intensity of this information exchange exceeds a certain threshold, "stormy activities" can occur, as for example during epileptic seizures in humans. Seizures are conditions that are characterized by episodes of uncontrolled electrical activity in the brain.

Symptoms

Seizures can impact any operation your brain coordinates. Symptoms differ depending on the kind of seizure; they may include:

- Inability to move
- Inability to speak
- Muscle jerking
- Sudden uncontrollable crying or laughter
- Uncontrollable blinking
- Uncontrollable limb shaking
- Visual and/or auditory hallucinations

Triggers

The factors that lead to seizures are often complex, unclear, and hard to pinpoint. Some common triggers for seizures are:

- Chemical imbalances
- Congenital conditions
- Genetic factors
- Infection
- Neurological problems
- Sleep deprivation

Benefits

The primary cannabinoid, THC, and cannabidiol have both been studied and found to have anti-convulsant properties in humans. A 2013 survey conducted by Porter and Jacobson showed that parents are using cannabidiol enriched cannabis for their children with epilepsy. The parents reported beneficial effects that included a reduction in seizure frequency, increased alertness, better mood, and improved sleep.

A number of people suffering from seizures have what is referred to as treatment-resistant seizures; not finding relief from conventional anti-convulsant drugs. It has been documented that cannabis has been used in treating these individuals with benefits, such as less frequent seizures, relaxing muscles, and as a sleeping aid.

Conventional Medicine

The conventional medication most frequently prescribed to treat partial-onset seizure is Aptiom (eslicarbazepine acetate). Although commonly prescribed to be taken alone or with other medication, this drug comes with a list of side effects; it may cause allergic reactions, liver problems, dizziness, nausea, nervous system problems, and suicidal behavior.

Medical Marijuana

Together with colleagues from the University of Mainz and teams from Heidelberg, Naples, and Madrid, researchers from the Max Planck Institute of Psychiatry in Munich showed that the brain's cannabinoid receptors together with the body's own cannabinoids constitute a system which protects the neurons from such hazardous excessive activities as seizures.

The researchers reported in the journal *Science* (October 3, 2002) that genetically modified mice lacking the cannabinoid receptor are highly susceptible to seizures and to concomitant cell death, for example the threshold for seizures is lower than in intact wild-type control mice (*see* Figure 2). Additionally, a drug-induced increase in the body's cannabinoids protects the brain from seizures, thus from resulting neuronal cell death.

The same brain machinery that responds to the active substance in marijuana provides "on-demand" protection against seizures.

In the brain, THC binds to proteins, called cannabinoid receptors, which act like an antenna and mediate the effects of THC. The existence of such an antenna has suggested that the brain produces cannabinoids on its own. In fact, such substances have been identified: they are fatty acid derivatives that can be released from neurons when needed. By binding to the cannabinoid receptor, both THC and endogenous cannabinoids change the neuron's reactivity to stimuli thus leading to a lowered transmission of electrical and chemical signals. THC and the body's cannabinoids are able to dampen the neuronal excitability.

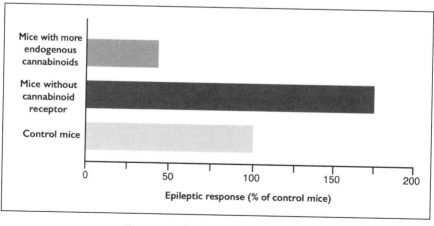

Figure 2. Epileptic Response in Mice

The researchers Dr. Ben Whalley, Dr. Gary Stephens, and Dr. Claire Williams, at their secret cannabis farm near London, have discovered that three compounds found in cannabis leaves can help to reduce and control seizures in epilepsy. Dr. Whalley, who is leading the research at the department of pharmacy at the University of Reading, said tests in animals have shown the marijuana compounds effective at preventing seizures and convulsions while also causing fewer side effects than existing epilepsy drugs.

There has been an appeal by the Epilepsy Foundation for increase to attainable medical marijuana and for increased research. It calls for restrictions made by the Drug Enforcement Administration (DEA) for clinical trials and research into medical marijuana for epilepsy to be lifted.

SKIN CANCER

See **CANCER.**

SKIN INFLAMMATION

See **INFLAMMATION.**

SLEEP DISORDERS

As reported by the National Sleep Foundation (NSF), almost six out of ten Americans chronicle having insomnia at least a few nights weekly. Insomnia is defined as an "inability to fall asleep or remain asleep long enough to feel rested, especially when the problem continues over time."

Sleep disorders are medical conditions in which sleep patterns are disrupted. Disruptions in sleep can obstruct the way you usually function physically, mentally, socially, and emotionally, and it can lead to serious consequences. Lack of sleep is a health concern because it can cause attention and memory problems, depressed mood, and body chemistry changes that foster heart disease, diabetes, and osteoporosis. As many as 47 million adults may be putting themselves at risk for injury and health and behavior problems because they aren't meeting their minimum need for sleep in order to be fully alert the next day. Sleep deprivation and sleep disorders are estimated to cost Americans over $100 billion annually

According to a 2008 survey of 1,137 employed U.S. adults, most Americans are losing sleep over news of a declining economy, increased cost of food and energy, rising unemployment, mortgage foreclosures, and plunging home values. The study said 9 of 10 respondents were losing sleep over economic turmoil. The vicious cycle of economic stress, lack of sleep, diminished immunity, and magnesium depletion is fully evident in the medical literature.

Symptoms

If you are experiencing any of the following signs of sleep deprivation on a regular basis, then you may be suffering from a sleep disorder.

- Difficulty concentrating
- Difficulty staying awake when sitting still, watching TV, or reading
- Emotional outbursts

- Fall asleep or feel very tired while driving
- Irritability or sleepiness during the day
- Napping daily
- Slow reactions

Benefits

Medical marijuana is an effective sleep aid because of its ability to relieve stress and provide physical relaxation. Studies have also shown that cannabis can promote a better quality of sleep, it can increase the duration of sleep, and help to regulate sleeping patterns.

Conventional Medicine

In an effort to combat sleep disorders, as many as 25 percent of the people in the United States use medications to help them sleep. More than half of all people aged 65 years and older have sleep problems. Yet, scientists have proven that poor sleep is not a natural part of aging.

The newest generation of sleep aids causes strange side effects, including sleepwalking and short-term amnesia. Ambien, the nation's best-selling prescription sleeping pill, shows up with regularity as a factor in traffic arrests, sometimes involving drivers who later say they were sleep-driving and have no memory of taking the wheel after taking the drug.

Steven Wells quit using the drug Ambien after becoming concerned about several episodes in which he woke up to find he had messily raided the refrigerator or in which he tore a towel rack out of a wall. We find none of these side effects from marijuana.

A patient with PTSD who takes marijuana and now shuns the array of medicines and sleeping pills she took because of the side effects is quoted as saying:

"If you take sleeping pills, you will bring yourself into sleep mode, you will succeed in getting yourself into bed and shutting off the light, but in the morning you are not the same person. You don't function. The quantity of pills I need in order to fall asleep will turn me into a zombie the next day. My brain is erased; people speak to me but I don't function. How can you live like that? How can you work like that, study, go out of the house, communicate with people?"

Medical Marijuana and Magnesium

What many want to know is why do we need cannabis when magnesium does the trick by itself? It seems that we are better off not taking any psychoactive drug if we can get the same benefit from a non-psychoactive drug. It would be perhaps safest to use magnesium first and then add marijuana when the reasons for lack of sleep are manifesting in hyper-acute symptoms that are not relieved by magnesium alone. Anyone who has ever used marijuana for any reason knows and understands the answer to the above question.

Medical marijuana. Though magnesium does reduce stress, depression, and restlessness in bed, it does not directly affect the mind, emotions, and spirit in a way that is easily detectable, whereas THC-laden cannabis does so most powerfully and instantly.

In September of 2010 the *New York Times* reported that, "People with chronic pain who took just a puff of marijuana three times a day got some mild pain relief and, with rare exceptions, did so without getting high, a Canadian study reports. (Yes, they inhaled.) The patients who suffered from persistent nerve damage and did not respond to other pain drugs also reported better sleep and less anxiety, the researchers said."

Magnesium. Animals placed on magnesium-deficient diets will commonly develop disorganized sleep and periods of wakefulness showing that magnesium deficiency is one of the root causes of sleep disturbances. Insomnia is one of the central, or neurotic, symptoms of chronic magnesium deficiency. A number of parasomnias (night terrors, nocturnal verbal and motor automatisms, and restless leg syndrome) are highly correlated to magnesium deficiency. When we lose magnesium we lose sleep, and then we lose our balance emotionally and then even depression or even hyperactivity can set in.

Sleep problems occur more frequently in adults as they age, making it increasingly difficult to deal with stress. Magnesium supplementation partially reverses age-related sleep abnormalities. Magnesium is an essential mineral that plays a major role in the functioning of the musculoskeletal system. Magnesium allows the muscles to relax providing a calming effect that allows for deeper relaxation and better sleep. Magnesium has a calming effect on the nervous system and is considered the "anti-stress" mineral and a natural tranquilizer.

Magnesium deficiency in children is characterized by excessive fidgeting, anxious restlessness, psychomotor instability, and learning difficulties in the presence of normal IQ.

—DR. MILDRED SEELIG.

In the elderly, magnesium supplements were found to improve sleep by decreasing the release of cortisol, a known cause of sleep disruption. Stress depletes magnesium and magnesium relieves stress. When your magnesium levels are low, your nervous system gets out of balance, and you feel on edge, naturally resulting in tightening muscles. *When we are under stress, our need for magnesium skyrockets.*

Chronic mental or physical stress serves as a trigger for heart attack or stroke. A study of college students, sleep deprived while studying for final exams, found that stress cut the concentration of magnesium in red blood cells in half and impaired the ability of blood vessels to widen (dilate) to control blood pressure. Lack of sleep can lead to chronic fatigue, which is associated with sudden-death heart attack. Chronically sleep-deprived adults commonly develop magnesium shortages that are also associated with a tendency for blood cells to clot, which is what causes strokes and heart attacks.

Several studies show a lack of magnesium can alter electrical activity in the brain, causing agitated sleep and frequent awakenings.

Sleep disorders caused by magnesium deficiency are usually agitated with frequent nocturnal awakenings. Magnesium helps people fall asleep faster and stay asleep.

According to the National Sleep Foundation, approximately 70 million people in the United States are affected with sleeping disorders. Approximately 12 million Americans have restless leg syndrome, a sleep and movement disorder characterized by unpleasant feelings (tingling, crawling, creeping and/or pulling) in the legs, resulting in an urge to move in order to relieve the symptoms.

People with poor quality sleep or sleep deprivation exhibit increased levels of interleukin-6 (IL6), the chemical that causes inflammation throughout the body. According to Dr. J. Durlach, the biological clock and magnesium status are linked, and a balanced magnesium status is important for the function of the mysterious pineal gland. Dr. Durlach sees the psycholeptic sedative effects of darkness amplified by magnesium. There probably is a strong relationship between melatonin and magnesium; certainly relative amounts of light and darkness affect the pineal gland and its production of melatonin.

> *Magnesium supplementation is usually helpful for relieving restless leg syndrome (RLS) and for treating insomnia.*

In a study by Dr. W. Davis, MD, 99 percent of his patients who used magnesium chloride as a means of combating insomnia experienced rapidly-induced and uninterrupted sleep. He also reported that waking tiredness disappeared and anxiety and tension diminished during the day for these patients.

Simply put, there is nothing like a hot soak in a magnesium chloride bath before bed. Such soaks are heaven on earth for people who suffer from insomnia and the feelings of restlessness in the limbs. Instead of ingesting further chemical toxins in the form of pharmaceutical sleeping pills, which further deteriorate health, one bathes in a deep relaxing hot magnesium bath similar to what is available at some of the most famous spas around the world. Not only will you sleep better but your entire health will be elevated. All one has to do is pour in some magnesium chloride. Nothing could be simpler except that one should also put in a pound of sodium bicarbonate and some sodium thiosulfate, especially if there is any chlorine in your bath water.

SPASMS

See **RESTLESS LEG SYNDROME and SEIZURES.**

SPINAL CORD INJURY/DISEASE

A spinal cord injury (damage or trauma to any part of the spinal cord or nerves at the end of the spinal canal) or disease often results in loss of motion, neuropathic pain, muscle spasms, loss of bladder control, erectile dysfunction, and depression.

Symptoms

Any type of spinal cord injury may generate one or more of the following symptoms:

- Breathing difficulty
- Loss of automatic activity
- Loss of bladder control
- Loss of bowel control
- Loss of function
- Loss of reflex function
- Loss of sensation
- Muscle spasms
- Pain
- Paralysis
- Sensitivity to stimuli
- Sexual dysfunction

Benefits

Researchers have confirmed medical marijuana's effectiveness in:

- Increasing appetite
- Reducing muscle spasms and spasticity
- Reducing pain
- Sleep disorders
- Suppressing muscle jerks

Conventional Medicine

Drugs may be prescribed for the initial injury and for the minor conditions that may emerge after the spinal cord injury. Initially, anti-inflammatory drugs, corticosteroids, may be administered followed by muscle relaxants, anti-depressants, and pain killers to combat the challenges stemming from a spinal cord injury.

Medical Marijuana

Various studies show that THC brings its own medical usefulness in treating spinal cord injuries. It improves the symptoms associated with the disorder and new research points to the possibility of cannabis compounds rehabilitating nerve function and growth of new cells.

SPORTS INJURY

An injury is considered to be a sports injury when it occurs while an athlete is participating in sports or exercising. A sports injury most often is a result of an accident, inadequate equipment, overuse of a body part, and poor training practices. The most common sports injuries are fractures, sprains and strains, knee injuries, shin splints, and dislocations.

Symptoms

The common warning signs and symptoms of a sports injury are:

- Heat
- Inflammation
- Loss of function
- Pain
- Redness
- Swelling

Benefits

Medical-grade cannabis has been shown to:

- Aid in sleeping disorders
- Reduce pain
- Reduce swelling and inflammation

Conventional Medicine

After experiencing a sports injury, pharmaceuticals, such as acetaminophens, NSAIDs and/or muscle relaxants, may be recommended to suppress pain and/or inflammation. NSAIDs, however, can inflame the stomach and cause bleeding. The over-prescription of opiods for sport injuries has lead to addiction problems and it is not limited to only professional sports.

Medical Marijuana

Multiple sports athletes have experienced positive benefits from the use of medical marijuana to treat sport injuries. The medicinal compounds in cannabis, THC and CBD, have been proven to decrease inflammation and control chronic pain and act as a muscle relaxant.

STRESS

It is no secret that the psychosocial state of a person does have a direct impact on the immune system. Stress has many different effects on the endocrine systems, including the fight or flight response (acute stress) with its activation of the sympathetic adrenal-medullary (SAM) system, the hypothalamic-pituitary-adrenocortical (HPAC) system, and other endocrine systems. The capabilities of the immune system are diminished after frequent activation of the autonomic nervous system in the case of chronic stress from sensory overload. Life is much more stressful when our basic needs go unmet.

Doctors should never lose sight of the fact that the endocrine system has close interactions with the immune system. Psychoneuroimmunology (PNI) incorporates facets of psychology, immunology, and neurosciences. It's a systems science that wraps its perceptions around landscapes of pathology.

> *Chronic stress can intensify inflammation and increase a person's risk for developing central nervous system infections, neurodegenerative diseases, like multiple sclerosis (MS), and other inflammatory diseases.*
>
> —AMERICAN PSYCHOLOGICAL ASSOCIATION, HARVARD HEALTH

Symptoms

Stress symptoms can impact your body, your thoughts, feelings, and behavior. If left unmanaged, the following stress symptoms can lead to a number of health problems.

- Angry outbursts
- Anxiety
- Change in sex drive
- Chest pain
- Depression
- Drug or alcohol abuse
- Exercising less often
- Fatigue
- Feeling overwhelmed
- Feeling sad
- Headache
- Irritability or anger
- Lack of motivation or focus
- Loss of appetite
- Muscle tension or pain
- Overeating
- Restlessness
- Sleep problems
- Social withdrawal
- Stomach upset

Triggers

In order to regulate and work at relieving your stress, you need to identify the source of your stress, such as:

- Beliefs
- Environment
- Fears
- Lack of control
- Major life changes
- Social
- Uncertainty
- Unpredictable events
- Workplace

Benefits

Research has demonstrated that cannabis and its derivatives are effective in reducing anxiety and relieving stress. It has been shown to be a natural option for dealing with the pressures of everyday life without the side effects of alcohol or drugs.

Conventional Medicine

Selective serotonin reuptake inhibitors (SSRIs) are the most commonly prescribed medications for anti-anxiety and anti-stress. These medications have some significant downsides. You can develop a physiological dependency and/or a psychological dependency. You can also experience possible side effects, including dry mouth, drowsiness, nausea, insomnia, restlessness, and sexual problems.

Medical Marijuana and Magnesium

A complete medical approach for stress should always include magnesium and might often include marijuana because it gives instant relief from most forms of stress.

Marijuana. Marijuana is a wonder drug for stress for it is able to soothe people's hurts and disturbed feelings safely and quickly. Medical marijuana offers great mental and emotional relief and makes people tranquil and less uptight. It is rare to see someone high on cannabinoids as edgy, irritable, easily startled, or on guard unless they also have a severe magnesium deficiency. Marijuana is just great at making people relax and feel better. During crises it allows people to divest their pains and fears. Marijuana simply makes stress more bearable; it is a highly useful medical tool.

Magnesium. Magnesium makes a perfect partner to cannabis for it gets down to the root of stress. A marginal deficiency of magnesium can easily be transformed into a more significant problem when stressful events trigger additional magnesium loss. In the extreme situations, stressful events trigger sudden drops of serum magnesium, leading to cardiac arrest. Magnesium is considered the "anti-stress" mineral. It is a natural tranquilizer that functions to relax skeletal muscles, as well as the smooth muscles of blood vessels and the gastrointestinal tract.

Even a mild deficiency of magnesium can cause increased sensitivity to noise, nervousness, irritability, mental depression, confusion, twitching, trembling, apprehension, and insomnia. Magnesium deficiency is generally characterized by the declining ability to respond to stress, increasing homeostatic imbalance, and increased risk of disease. It is widely researched and recognized that magnesium deficiency commonly occurs in critical illness and correlates with a higher mortality and worse clinical outcomes in the intensive care unit (ICU).

Research published in the American Journal of Epidemiology *in 2002 shows that when the diets of 2,566 children ages 11 to 19 were studied, less than 14 percent of boys and 12 percent of girls had adequate intakes of magnesium.*

While stress leads to magnesium depletion, magnesium deficiency causes stress-related symptoms, such as insomnia, muscle tension, migraines, and irritability. You can avoid this vicious cycle by staying on top of your magnesium needs. Climb into a warm *magnesium bath* and feel the tensions slip away from your body and soul. It will simply help you cope. And don't forget to eat some good chocolate; it too is very high in magnesium; mood control is the main reason people eat chocolate.

Mg deficiency increases susceptibility to the physiologic damag produced by stress. The adrenergic effects of psychological stress induce a shift of Mg from the intracellular to the extracellular space, increasing urinary excretion and eventually depleting body stores.

—Dr. Leo Galland

In recent years we've seen an increase of all kinds of weird violence as magnesium levels are driven lower and lower. Police Chief Nannette H. Hegerty of Milwaukee said a few years ago that, "We're seeing a very angry population, and they don't go to fists anymore, they go right to guns," she said. "When we ask, 'Why did you shoot this guy?' it's, 'He bumped into me.' or, 'He looked at my girl the wrong way.'" said Police Commissioner Sylvester M. Johnson of Philadelphia. "It's not like they're riding around doing drive-by shootings. It's arguments—stupid arguments over stupid things." While arguments have always made up a large number of homicides, the police say the trigger point now comes faster. In robberies, Milwaukee's Chief Hegerty said, "Even after the person gives up, the guy with the gun shoots him anyway. We didn't have as much of that before."

There is little question that stress can kill and magnesium deficiencies may very well be the underlying cause of this stress. Harvard physiologist Walter Cannon recognized 90 years ago that when confronted by a threat—physical or emotional, real or imagined—the body responds with a rise in blood pressure, heart rate, muscle tension, and breathing rate. We now know that this physiological "stress response" involves hormones and inflammatory chemicals that can, when overdosed, foster everything from headaches to heart attacks.

> *Magnesium deficiency causes serotonin deficiency with possible resultant aberrant behaviors, including depression, suicide, or irrational violence.*
>
> —PAUL MASON

It is clear that magnesium deficiency or imbalance plays a role in the symptoms of mood disorders. Observational and experimental studies have shown an association between magnesium and aggression, anxiety, ADHD, bipolar disorder, depression, and schizophrenia.

> *Patients who had made suicide attempts (by using either violent or nonviolent means) had significantly lower mean CSF magnesium level irrespective of the diagnosis.*

STROKE

A stroke has an effect on the arteries leading to the brain and the arteries within the brain. When an artery that carries oxygen and nutrients to the brain is blocked by a clot or when the artery ruptures a stroke will occur. It is a quick loss of brain function caused by an absence of blood flow.

Symptoms

Often the symptoms appear without warning followed by a stroke. The common symptoms are:

- Confusion
- Difficulty seeing
- Difficulty walking
- Dizziness
- Headache
- Numbness or paralysis in face, arm, or leg (usually on the same side of body)
- Slurred speech

Triggers

A number of factors can elevate your risk of a stroke. Your chances are increased if the following conditions exist:

- Being overweight or obese
- Cardiovascular disease
- Cigarette smoking
- Diabetes
- Drinking heavily
- High blood pressure
- High cholesterol
- Lack of exercise
- Sleep apnea
- Using illicit drugs

Family history of stroke, age, race, and gender may also increase the risk.

Benefits

There is evidence that the most common cannabinoids, THC and CBD, can reduce the inflammation that is brought upon by a stroke. In addition, the cannibinoids are also presumed to reduce brain damage by heightening the survival of neurons.

Conventional Medicine

Commonly anticoagulant medicines and antiplatelet medicines to prevent blood clots are recommended, as well as cholesterol and blood pressure lowering medicines. Blood thinning medications, such as warfarin, may cause bleeding from the gums after brushing, diarrhea, vomiting, or fever. Statins, used to lower cholesterol levels, may result in headaches, nausea, vomiting, abdominal pain, dizziness, bloating, diarrhea, muscle aches, or a rash.

Medical Marijuana

THC and cannabidiol provide equal defense against cell damage. Cannabis contains a chemical that can protect cells by acting as an antioxidant.

In test-tube experiments, researchers at the National Institutes of Health (NIH) in Bethesda, Maryland exposed rat nerve cells to a toxin that is typically released during strokes. Cannabidiol reduces the extent of damage researchers reported to the National Academy of Sciences. More effective than vitamins C or E, strong antioxidants, such as cannabidiol will neutralize free radicals and so might limit the damage and reduce the severity of ischemic strokes.

A study at the University of Arizona in Tucson turned up no side effects of cannabidiol in people given large doses. This is a promising area of research particularly since we have so few effective means of treating neurological damages.

TOURETTE SYNDROME

Tourette syndrome (TS) is a chronic, in many cases, inherited neuropsychiatric disorder characterized by the presence of multiple physical tics, motor and vocal. Tics are involuntary movements or sounds that are rapid and repeated.

Symptoms

The symptoms, as follow, extend from mild to severe, and the length of time they last can vary.

- Abnormal sleep disturbances
- Anxiety
- Body twisting
- Coughing
- Depression
- Eye blinking
- Facial tics
- Foot stamping

- Head jerking
- Motor Tics
- Neck stretching
- Obsessive compulsive thoughts
- Repeated involuntary movements
- Throat clearing tics
- Uncontrollable vocal sounds

Triggers

The factors leading to Tourette syndrome are basically unknown, however genetics plays a role in many cases. It is believed that environmental and developmental factors may also play a role.

Benefits

There have been several research studies citing the benefit of treating TS with cannabis.

- Acts as a sleeping aid
- Helps with depression

- Reduces symptoms
- Reduces tics

Conventional Medicine

Medications that are generally prescribed to control or reduce the symptoms that are associated with Tourette's, they include ADHD medications, Botox injections, antidepressants, antiseizure drugs, and medication that block or lessen dopamine; at present there is no cure. As with most medications, there are potential negative side effects.

Medical Marijuana

Although the use of cannabis to treat TS is still not officially approved, studies have shown that THC, the "active ingredient" in marijuana, is recognized in decreasing tics without any side effects.

The *New York Times* published the following: "There's one thing that helps my Tourette's more than anything, and it's marijuana," says Louis Centanni. Dr. Robert A. King and Dr. James F. Leckman of the Yale School of Medicine believe that clinical studies have shown that marijuana can be effective in relieving the symptoms of this disease. "A number of individuals with severe Tourette's regularly use marijuana and report that it calms them and eases their tics. And a few randomized clinical trials of delta 9-tetrahydrocannabinol, or THC, the active ingredient in marijuana, have been carried out." Controlled research on treating Tourette syndrome with a synthetic version of THC showed that patients had a beneficial response without serious adverse effects.

Dr. William Dale, section chief of geriatrics and palliative medicine at the University of Chicago Medical Center, said marijuana *raises users' heart rates and lowers their blood pressure*. Natural Allopathic Medicine mixes magnesium chloride in a protocol with cannabinoids to compete for the supreme medical choice of doctors who are struggling to keep their patients' blood pressure and stress levels down while simultaneously strengthening the heart with the extra help of iodine.

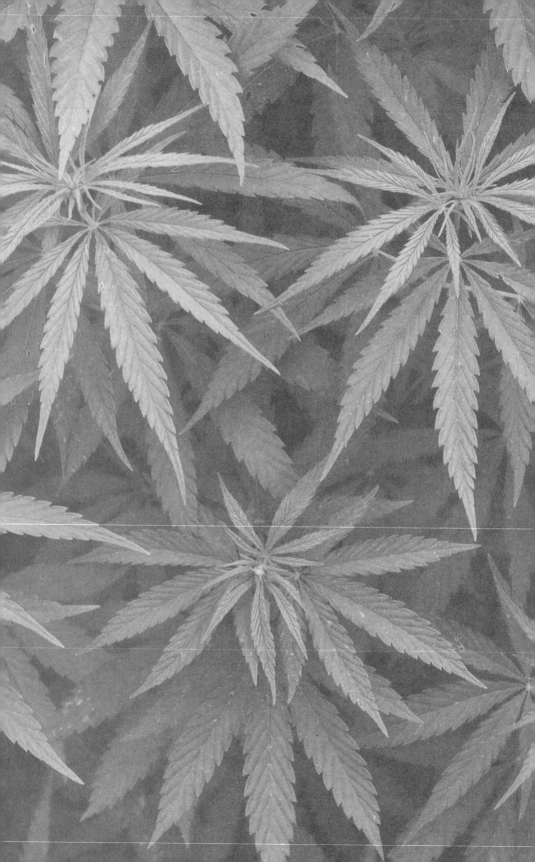

Conclusion

Hundreds of thousands of people around the world die every year from *properly* prescribed pharmaceuticals taken as recommended. In the United States alone, the number is over 100,000 deaths per year. On the other hand, millions of others around the world use cannabis for medical purposes without *one single death* being officially attributed to the use of marijuana.

As the facts show, mainstream medicine needs to add cannabinoids in its fight against cancer, diabetes, heart disease, and neurological diseases, as well as stress and emotional upset. By incorporating cannabinoids into our medical practices we can allow physical medicine to have a greater and more profound impact on emotional medicine and psychology. All it takes is to have our doctors and other healthcare professionals broaden their horizons by learning about and making use of this valuable modality.

As with any effective medicine there are warnings, precautions, and contraindications. It is always important to use any medicinal wisely. Nevertheless, at this point in human civilization, the cannabis plant offers a huge helping hand to our race at a time of great need.

In my book's Introduction, I mentioned that there is a revolution going on in expanding the legal use of marijuana. It is a fight that has gone on for years, however now we are seeing change—now more and more people are able to legal use this wondrous plant. And I am happy to report that the changes in our state laws are a direct result of our citizens making themselves heard. However, the bad news is that there are still powerful forces out there that continue to hold back the use of one of nature's most effective plants. With the influence exerted by the pharmaceutical industry on the medical community, the use of cannabinoids still remains out of reach for millions.

In closing, I hope you find the information in this book helpful, and I also hope you realize that not only do you have a powerful resource in your hands, but you also have the power in your hands to make important changes—in the health community and in the law.

Resources

The resources below have been set up to provide information for those interested in understanding how medical marijuana may be used within their states. As time goes on more states will be legalizing the use of medical marijuana and should also have resources available for their state residents. Please note all information below may be subject to change. It is therefore important to contact these centers before planning a visit.

MEDICAL MARIJUANA RESOURCE CENTERS AND DISPENSARIES

By State

For residents of **Alaska:**
Alaska Cannabis Club
Provides safe access to a wide variety of medication, dried herbs, medibles, and concentrates, as well as a staff with extensive experience in medical cannabis provisions.

628 Gambell Street
Anchorage, AK 99501
(907) 227-6418
www.akcannabisclub.com

For residents of **Arizona:**
Sunflower Meds
Trained staff to help you achieve the best quality of life possible by providing an alternative, medical marijuana, rather than expensive and often addictive drugs.

Sunflower Meds Phoenix
10827 S 51st Street #104
Phoenix, AZ 850044
(480) 350-7624
www.sunflowermeds.com

Sunflower Meds Mesa
5205 E. University Drive
Mesa, AZ 85205
(480) 500-5054
www.sunflowermeds.com

For residents of **California:**
United Patient Group
A resource center that helps medical marijuana users of all levels feel comfortable.

336 Bon Air Center, #361
Greenbrae, CA 94904
(415) 524-8099
www.info@unitedpatientsgroup.com

For residents of **Colorado:**
Trichome Health Consultants
Provides an educated staff to inform and answer questions as well as a medical marijuana dispensary.

2117 W Colorado Avenue
Colorado Springs, CO 80904
(719) 635-6337
www.thcmed.com

For residents of **Connecticut:**
The Healing Corner
Professionals work with patients to determine their individual needs and prescribe the proper type of medical marijuana.

159 East Main Street
Bristol, CT 06010
(860) 583-HEAL (4325)
www.thehealingcorner.com

For residents of **Delaware:**
First State Compassion Center
Provides certified patients with safe, affordable access to high quality medical cannabis in a dignified, compassionate environment.

37 Germany Drive
Wilmington, DE 19804
(302) 543-2100
www.allbud.com/dispensaries/
    delaware/wilmington/first-state-
    compassion-center

For residents of **Hawaii:**
Big Island Dispensary
Provides medical marijuana for a variety of illnesses.

Locations in Kona, Hilo, and Pahoa.
www.bigislanddispensary.com/

For residents of **Illinois:**
The Healing Clinic
A medical cannabis patient advocacy center offering integrative primary care.

Lakeview
1443 W. Belmont Avenue
Chicago, IL 60657
(312) 890-6113
(844) 249-5580
www.info@thehealingclinic.org

Highland Park
322 Skokie Valley Road #104
Highland Park, IL 60035
(312) 890-6113
(844) 249-5580
www.info@thehealingclinic.org

Flossmoor
3235 Vollmer Road #139
Flossmoor, IL 60422
(312) 890-6113
(844) 249-5580
www.info@thehealingclinic.org

For residents of **Maine:**
Wellness Connection
Experts provide answers to your wellness needs and medical cannabis needs.

67 Center Street
Bath, ME 04530
(207) 354-4455
www.info@mainewellness.org

For residents of **Massachusetts:**
Patriot Care
Provides medical marijuana services
and products for qualifying patients.

21 Milk Street
Boston, MA
(617) 500-1375
https://patriotcare.org/

70 Industrial Avenue
Lowell, MA
(978) 289-1088
https://patriotcare.org/

For residents of **Michigan:**
Green Planet
Provides knowledgeable medical
cannabis consultants and a range of
medical cannabis.

700 Tappan Avenue
Ann Arbor, MI 48104
(734) 845-2172
www.info@greenpaneta2.org

For residents of **Minnesota:**
Leafline Labs
Provides a range of medical cannabis
options tailored to your condition.

Eagan
2795 Pilot Knob Road
Eagan, MN 55121
(651) 846-9245
www.infro@leaflinelabs.com

St. Cloud
141 33rd Avenue South
St. Cloud, MN 56301
(320) 443-6250
www.infro@leaflinelabs.com

Saint Paul
550Vandalia Street
Saint Paul, MN 55114
www.infro@leaflinelabs.com

For residents of **Montana:**
Lionheart
Provides a knowledgeable staff and
high quality medical cannabis.

1117 N 7th Avenue
Bozeman, MT 59715
(844) 586-2837
www.info@lionheartcaregiving.com

For residents of **Nevada:**
Nevada Medical Marijuana
Provides a knowledgeable staff and
quality state regulated and tested
medical cannabis.

3195 St. Rose Parkway, Suite #212
Henderson, NV
(702) 298-4820
www.nevadamedicalmarijuana.com

For residents of **New Hampshire:**
Sanctuary Alternative Treatment
Center
Provides therapeutic cannabis to
help ease pain from more than 14
conditions. Evaluations, dietary
considerations, and comfort level
directs patients to a full range of
medication options.

658 Tenney Mountain Highway
Plymouth, NH 03264
(603) 346-4619
www.sanctuaryatc.org

For residents of **New Jersey: Breakwater Treatment & Wellness** Consultants help you find the medical cannabis that is engineered to treat your specific condition or disease.

2 Corporate Drive
Suite E
Cranbury, NJ 08512
(732) 703-7300
www.breakwateratc.com/

For residents of **New Mexico: New Mexico Brief Relief— Medical Cannabis Consultants** This program allows the beneficial use of medical cannabis in a regulated system for debilitating medical conditions and medical treatments.

4730 Pan American Fwy NE, Ste E
Albuquerque, MN 87109
(505) 433-1773

For residents of **New York State: Medical Marijuana Consultants** Provides answers to which conditions are New York State approved conditions and contacts may help you fit your diagnosis into one of the qualifying conditions. Also lists New York State medical marijuana dispensaries.

4000 Medical Center Drive, Suite 217
Fayetteville, NY 13066
(844) 333-7639
(315) 637-7900
Fax: (315) 637-7907
www.medmarijuanaconsultants.com

For the residents of **Oregon: Cherry City Compassion Medical/ Recreational Marijuana** Provides a compassionate and knowledgeable staff and quality medical cannabis treatment.

2025 25th Street SE
Salem, OR 97302
(971) 273-7607
www.cherrycitycompasion.com

For residents of **Rhode Island: Medical Cannabis Consultants** Consists of a team of health care professionals that provide alternative therapeutic options.

610 Ten Rod Road
North Kingston, RI 02852
(401) 667-7778
www.thegreenscript.com

For residents of **Vermont: Southern Vermont Wellness** Offers cannabis treatments and alternative health practices as supplements to standardized medicine.

1222 Putney Road
Brattleboro, VT 05303
(844) 789-9333
www.cvdvt.org/

For residents of the state of **Washington: Washington State Department of Health** A list of medically endorsed marijuana stores that have at least one certified medical marijuana consultant on staff.

(800) 525-0127
www.doh.wa.gov/Portals/1/
    Documents/Pubs/608017.pdf

Hemp and Cannabis Foundation
Provides a guide to finding doctors
or clinics that specializes in medical
marijuana recommendations
throughout the country.
71 Columbia Street
Suite 300
Seattle, WA 98104
(855) 4-Leafly
www.leafly.com/news/health/how-
    to-find-a-doctor-or-clinic-that-
    specializes-in-medical-mariju

25 Legal Medical Marijuana States
    and DC
A list of states that have legalized
the use of the marijuana plant for
medical purposes.
Email: http://medicalmarijuana
    .procon.org/view.resource.php?
    resourceID=000881

Leafly
Provides a listing of medical
marijuana dispensaries in the United
States. In addition, information to
help you find the ideal edible,
concentrate, or topical cannabis
strain.
(855) 4-Leafly
www.leafly.com

MEDICAL MARIJUANA DOSING

Americans For Safe Access
Provides a guide for using medical
cannabis safely.

Offices in Oakland, Los Angeles,
and Washington, DC
(202) 857-4272
www.info@safeaccessnow.org

CanniMed
Provides recommended dosing
and delivery methods of medical
cannabis based on the type and
severity of your condition and the
delivery method you choose.

1 Plant Technology Road
Box 19A, RR#5
Saskatoon, SK
Canada, S7K 3J8
(855) 787-1577

Fax: (844) 231-8929
www.info@cannimed.com

Medicinal Marijuana Association
Provides the potency of a variety of
cannabis types and recommended
proper dosage of medical cannabis
and delivery methods.

120 Adelaide Street West
Suite 2500
Toronto, Ontario
M5H1T1
(855) 420-8222
www.medicinalmarijuanaassociation.
com/medical-marijuana-blog

ProCon.org
Provides proper dosage recommendations and how you can control the dose.

233 Wilshire Blvd.
Suite 200
Santa Monica, CA 90401
(310) 451-9596
http://medicalmarijuana.procon.org/
    view.answers

COOKING WITH CANNABIS

Cooking With Cannabis 101
A guide to cooking with cannabis:
extraction methods, decarboxylation,
and how to calculate THC when
cooking with cannabis. The website
provides simple starter recipes as
well.
http://herb.co/cooking-with-
    cannabis

The Cannabist
Recipe: Extracting Cannabis into Oil
or Butter
www.thecannabist.co/2014/02/03/
    kitchen-kush-making-canna-oils-
    recipe/3451

MARIJUANA-BASED TINCTURES

Southern Cannabis
How to make cannabis infused
    vegetable glycerin
https://www.southerncannabis.org/c
    ooking-with-cannabis/cannabis-
    vegetable-glycerin/

Cannabis Tinctures 101
What are they, how to make them,
    and how to use them
www.leafly.com/news/cannabis-
    101/cannabis-tinctures-101-what-
    are-they-how-to-make-them-and-
    how-to

HEMP OIL

Rick Simpson's Medicinal Hemp Oil
How to make Rick Simpson's
    medicinal hemp oil safely. -
    YouTube
https://www.youtube.com/watch?v
    =KZXGH6mYr3Y

MAGNESIUM

Magnesium Online Library
Magnesium For Health Foundation
Editor, Paul Mason
P.O. Box 1417
Patterson, CA 95363
www.mgwater.com

References

CHAPTER I. CANNABIS—THE HOLY HERB

Fishman, Rachelle HB. "Cannabis science: cannabinoid derivative protects neurons." *The Lancet.* Vol 348 (No. 9039) 1996 November 23. www.erowid.org/plants/cannabis/references/journal/1996_fishman_lancet_1/1996_fishman_lancet_1_text.shtml

Journal of the National Cancer Institute Advance Access. "Breakthrough discovered in medical marijuana cancer treatment." 2007 December 25.
http://salem-news.com/articles/january112008/cancer_treatment_11008.php

McAllister, Sean PhD. "THC and CBD enhances inhibitory effects on brain cancer." 2010 November 1.
www.cannabisni.com/medicinal-cannabis-news/1313-thc-and-cbd-enhances-inhibitory-effects-on-brain-cancer-

Miller, Kelli. "Marijuana chemical may fight brain cancer." *WebMD Health News* 2009 April 1. www.webmd.com/cancer/brain-cancer/news/20090401/marijuana-chemical-may-fight-brain-cancer

Zuardi AW. "Cannabidiol: from an inactive annabinoid to a drug with wide spectrum of action." *Revista Brasileria de Psiquiatria;* 2008 September 30;(3) :271–80.
www.ncbi.nlm.nih.gov/pubmed/18833429

CHAPTER 2. THE ESSENTIAL MEDICINE

Carey, Benedict. "Drugs to curb agitation are said to be ineffective for alzheimer's." *New York Times,* 2006 October 12.
www.nytimes.com/2006/10/12/health/12dementia.html?_r=1&th&emc=th&oref=slogin

Carter GT, Weydt P. "Cannabis: old medicine with new promise for neurological disorders." *Current Opinion Investigating Drugs* 2002 March;3(3) :437–40.

Carter GT and Rosen BS. Muscular Dystrophy Association (MDA) , Neuromuscular Disease Clinic, Department of Rehabilitation Medicine, University of Washington School of Medicine, Seattle, Washington, USA. *American Journal of Hospice and Palliative Care;* 18(4) :264–70 (ISSN: 1049-9091) .

Clinical Calcium"Magnesium and inflammation: lessons from animal models." 2005 Feb;15(2) :245–8. *Japanese Review* PMID: 15692164 [PubMed - indexed for MEDLINE].

DePedro-Cuesta J. "Studies on the prevalence of paralysis agitans by tracer methodology," *Acta Neurologica Scandinavica* 1987. Supplement 112, 75: 106.

Eljaschewitsch et al. "The Endogenous Cannabinoid Anandamide (AEA) protects neurons during CNS inflammation by induction of MKP-1 in microglial cells." *Publishing in Neuron* 49 2006 January; 567–79, DOI 10.1016/j.neuron.2005.11.027
www.neuron.org

Eubanks, Lisa M. PhD et al. "A molecular link between the active component of marijuana and alzheimer's disease pathology." *Molecular Pharmaceutics* 2006 August 9.

Fishman, Rachelle HB. "Cannabis science: cannabinoid derivative protects neurons." *The Lancet.* Vol 348 (No. 9039) 1996 November 23. www.erowid.org/plants/cannabis/references/journal/1996_fishman_lancet_1/1996_fishman_lancet_1_text.shtml

Foster, Harold D. PhD. "Parkinson's disease, multiple sclerosis, and amyotrophic lateral sclerosis: The iodine-dopachrome-glutamate hypothesis." *The Journal of Orthomolecular Medicine* Vol. 14, 3rd Quarter 1999.
http://orthomolecular.org/library/jom/1999/articles/1999-v14n03-p128.shtml

George Washington University, Department of Medicine. "Pathobiology of magnesium deficiency: a cytokine/neurogenic inflammation hypothesis." *American Journal of Physiology* 1992;263:R734–7.

Grotenhermen F, Russo EB, editors. "Cannabis and cannabinoids: pharmacology, toxicology, and therapeutic potential." Binghamton, New York: Haworth Press. p. 195–204.

Growing L et al. "Therapeutic use of cannabis: clarifying the debate." *Drug and Alcohol Review* (1998) 17: 445–452.

Independent Drug Monitoring Unit. "Cannabis and stress anxiety." 2016 October 17.
www.idmu.co.uk/canstressdepres.htm

Jacobsson, Stig OP, Wallin, Thomas and Fowler, Christopher J. "Inhibition of rat C6 glioma cell proliferation by endogenous and synthetic cannabinoids. Relative involvement of cannabinoid and vanilloid receptors." *Journal of Pharmacology and Experimental Therapeutics* Vol. 299, Issue 3, 2001 December, 299 (3) 951–959.

Journal of the National Cancer Institute Advance Access "Breakthrough discovered in medical marijuana cancer treatment" 2007 December 25. http://salem-news.com/articles/january112008/cancer_treatment_11008.php

Joy JE, Watson SJ and Benson JA. „Marijuana and medicine: assessing the science base institute of medicine". Washington, DC: National Academy Press; 1999.

Massi et al. "Antitumor effects of cannabidiol, a non-psychotropic cannabinoid, on human glioma cell lines." *Journal of Pharmacology and Experimental Therapeutics Fast Forward* 2004 308: 838–845.

Mazur A, Maier JA, Rock E, Gueux E, Nowacki W, Rayssiguier Y. "Magnesium and the inflammatory response." 2006 Apr 19. www.ncbi.nlm.nih.gov/entrez/query.fcgi?cmd=Retrieve&db=pubmed&dopt=Abstract&list_uids=16712775&itool=iconabstr&query_hl=2&itool=pubmed_docsum

McAllister, Sean PhD. "THC and CBD Enhances Inhibitory Effects on Brain Cancer." 2010 November 1.
www.cannabisni.com/medicinal-cannabis-news/1313-thc-and-cbd-enhances-inhibitory-effects-on-brain-cancer-

Medical News Today. "Marijuana's Active Ingredient May Slow Progression Of Alzheimer's Disease." 2006 October 1.
www.medilexicon.com/medicalnews.php?newsid=53664

Rubenowitz E, Axelsson G and Rylander R. "Magnesium and calcium in drinking water and death from acute myocardial infarction in women." *Epidemiology* 1999; 10:31–36.

Vinciguerra, Moore and Brennen, "Inhalation of marijuana as an anti-emetic for chemotherapy." *New York State Journal of Medicine* Vol. 88, pp. 525–527, 1988.

Wikipedia. Medical Cannabis.
http://en.wikipedia.org/wiki/Medical_cannabis#cite_note-usd-53
http://en.wikipedia.org/wiki/Medical_cannabis#cite_note-cbs-54

Zuardi AW. "Cannabidiol: from an inactive annabinoid to a drug with wide spectrum of action." *Revista Brasileria de Psiquiatria* 2008 September 30;(3) :271–80.
www.ncbi.nlm.nih.gov/pubmed/18833429

CHAPTER 3. SAFE FOR MEN, WOMEN, AND CHILDREN

Comstock G. "Water hardness and cardiovascular diseases." *American Journal of Epidemiology* 1979; 110:375–400.

Joshi, Mohit. "Periodontal disease causes gestational diabetes in pregnant women: study." 2008 March.
www.topnews.in/health/periodontal-disease-causes-gestational-diabetes-pregnant-women-study-21596

Marx A and Neutra R. "Magnesium in drinking water and ischemic heart disease." *Epidemiologic Review* 1997; 19:258–272

Meier, Barry. "A drug on trial: justice and science; boy's murder case entangled in fight over antidepressants." *New York Times* 2004 August 23.
www.nytimes.com/2004/08/23/business/23drug.html?th

Miller, Kelli. "Marijuana chemical may fight brain cancer." *WebMD Health News* 2009 April 1.
www.webmd.com/cancer/brain-cancer/news/20090401/marijuana-chemical-may-fight-brain-cancer

Penner, Elizabeth A. MD, MPH et al. "The Impact of Marijuana Use on Glucose, Insulin, and Insulin Resistance among US Adults." *The American Journal of Medicine;* Volume 126, Issue 7, Pages 583–589, July 2013.
www.amjmed.com/article/S0002-9343(13) 00200-3/abstract

Rubenowitz E, Axelsson G, Rylander R. "Magnesium and calcium in drinking water and death from acute myocardial infarction in women." *Epidemiology* 1999; 10:31–36.

CHAPTER 4. MEDICAL MARIJUANA IN PEDIATRIC MEDICINE

Journal Cancer Research. "Marijuana ingredient inhibits VEGF pathway required for brain tumor blood vessels." 2004 August 15.

www.eurekalert.org/pub_releases/2004-08/aafc-mii081204.php

Journal of the National Cancer Institute Advance Access. "Breakthrough discovered in medical marijuana cancer treatment." 2007 December 25.

http://salem-news.com/articles/january112008/cancer_treatment_11008.php

Miller, Kelli. "Marijuana chemical may fight brain cancer" *WebMD Health News* 2009 April 1. www.webmd.com/cancer/brain-cancer/news/20090401/marijuana-chemical-may-fight-brain-cancer

CHAPTER 5. THERAPEUTIC CANNABIS DOSAGES

Carey, Benedict. "Drugs to curb agitation are said to be ineffective for alzheimer's." *New York Times,* 2006 October 12. www.nytimes.com/2006/10/12/health/12dementia.html?_r=1&th&emc=th&oref=slogin

Conrad, Chris. "Cannabis yields and dosage." 2007. www.safeaccessnow.net/yieldsdosage.htm

Eubanks, Lisa M. PhD et al. "A molecular link between the active component of marijuana and alzheimer's disease pathology." *Molecular Pharmaceutics* 2006 August 9.

Independent Drug Monitoring Unit. "Cannabis and stress anxiety." 2016 October 13. www.idmu.co.uk/canstressdepres.htm

Medical News Today. "Marijuana's active ingredient may slow progression of alzheimer's disease." 2006 October 1. www.medilexicon.com/medicalnews.php?newsid=53664.

CHAPTER 6. TRANSDERMAL AND ORAL CANNABIS

Clinical Calcium."Magnesium and inflammation: lessons from animal models." 2005 Feb;15(2):245–8. *Japanese Review.* PMID: 15692164 [PubMed - indexed for MEDLINE]

Foster, Harold D. PhD. "Parkinson's disease, multiple sclerosis and amyotrophic lateral sclerosis: the iodine-dopachrome-glutamate hypothesis." *The Journal of Orthomolecular Medicine* Vol. 14, 3rd Quarter 1999. http://orthomolecular.org/library/jom/1999/articles/1999-v14n03-p128.shtml

Nature 434. "Low dose cannabinoid therapy reduces progression of atherosclerosis in mice." 2005 April 782–786. www.420magazine.com/forums/cannabinoid-receptors-cb2/148638-low-dose-oral-cannabinoid-therapy-reduces-progression-atherosclerosis-mice.html

CHAPTER 7. HEMP OIL

McNamee, David. "New health benefits associated with hempseed oil." *Medical News Today* 2014 February 1. www.medicalnewstoday.com/articles/272024.php

Natural Health 365. "Hemp oil effectively kills cancer cells." 2012 September 28. ww.naturalhealth365.com/hemp-oil.html/

Simpson, Rick. *Phoenix of Tears.* Amazon Digital Services, 2013 September 16.

Simpson, Rick. *Natures Answer for Cancer.* Amazon Digital Services, 2013 September 16.

The Health Cure. "Spain study confirms hemp oil cures cancer without side effects." 2013 March 3. www.thehealthcure.org/spain-study-confirms-hemp-oil-cures-cancer-without-side-effects/

CHAPTER 8. THE LAW

Armentano, Paul. *"Pot shows promise as cancer cure."* 2004 September 28.

www.alternet.org/drugreporter/20008/

Grinspoon, Lester. "The shifting medical view on marijuana" *Boston Globe* 2003 August 17- Editorial / Opinion Op-ed.

Growing L et al. "Therapeutic use of cannabis: clarifying the debate. Drug and Alcohol." *Review* (1998) , 17: 445–452.

www.redorbit.com/news/health/1259095/doctor_group_endorses_medical_marijuana/

National Organziation for the Reform of Marijuana Laws. "Cannabinoids as cancer hope."

http://norml.org/component/zoo/category/cannabinoids-as-cancer-hope

Scannell, Kate. "Bush's painful obsession with medical pot." *Oakland Tribune* 2003 October 26.

PART 2

American Psychological Association "How Chronic Stress Worsens." 2007 August 20.

Amtmann D, Weydt P, Johnson KL, Jensen MP, and Carter GT. „Survey of cannabis use in patients with amyotrophic lateral sclerosis." *American Journal of Hospital Palliative Care* 2004;21:95–104.

Brainard J. "Marijuana chemical tapped to fight strokes." *Science News* Vol. 154, No. 2, 1998 July 11, p. 20.

California Pacific Medical Center Research Institute. "THC and CBD enhances inhibitory effects on brain cancer." 2010 January 6.

Carey, Benedict. "Drugs to curb agitation are said to be ineffective for alzheimer's," *New York Times,* 2006 October 12.

Carter GT and Weydt P. "Cannabis: old medicine with new promise for neurological disorders." *Current Opinion Investigating Drugs* 2002 Mar;3(3) :437–40.

Clinical Calcium."Magnesium and inflammation: lessons from animal models." 2005 Feb;15(2) :245–8. Review. Japanese. PMID: 15692164 [PubMed - indexed for MEDLINE]

Comstock G. "Water hardness and cardiovascular diseases." *American Journal of Epidemiology* 1979; 110:375–400.

DePedro-Cuesta J. "Studies on the prevalence of Paralysis Agitans by tracer methodology," *Acta Neurologica Scandinavica,* 1987. Supplement 112, 75: 106

Eljaschewitsch et al.: "The Endogenous Cannabinoid Anandamide (AEA) protects neurons during CNS inflammation by induction of MKP-1 in microglial cells." *Publishing in Neuron 49,* 2006 January 5; 67–79, DOI 10.1016/j.neuron.2005.11.027. www.neuron.org

Eubanks, Lisa M., PhD et al. "A molecular link between the active component of marijuana and alzheimer's disease pathology" *Molecular Pharmaceutics* 2006 August 9.

Foster, Harold D. PhD. "Parkinson's disease, multiple sclerosis and amyotrophic lateral sclerosis: the iodine-dopachrome-glutamate hypothesis." *The Journal of Orthomolecular Medicine* Vol. 14, 3rd Quarter 1999.

Franklin, Deborah. "Poisonings from a propular pain reliever are rising." *The New York Times* 2005 November 29.

George Washington University, Department of Medicine. "Pathobiology of magnesium deficiency: a cytokine/neurogenic inflammation hypothesis." *American Journal of Physiology* 1992;263:R734-7.

Hashimoto T, Nishi K, Nagasao J, Tsuji S, and Oyanagi Kin Res. "Magnesium exerts both preventive and ameliorating effects in an in vitro rat Parkinson disease model involving 1-methyl-4-phenylpyridinium (MPP+) toxicity in dopaminergic neurons." 2008 Mar 4;1197:143–51.

Journal Cancer Research. "Marijuana ingredient inhibits VEGF pathway required for brain tumor blood vessels." 2004 August 15.

Journal of Neuroscience. "Prevention of Alzheimer's disease pathology by cannabinoids: neuroprotection mediated by blockage of microglial activation." 2005 February 23.

Journal of the National Cancer Institute Advance Access. "Breakthrough discovered in medical marijuana cancer treatment." 2007 December 25.

Kimball ES, Schneider CR, Wallace NH and Hornby PJ. "Agonists of cannabinoid receptor 1 and 2 inhibit experimental colitis induced by oil of mustard and by dextran sulfate sodium." *American Journal of Physiology-Gastrointestinal and Liver Physiology* 2006 Mar 30.

Massi et al. "Antitumor effects of cannabidiol, a non-psychotropic cannabinoid, on human glioma cell lines." *Journal of Pharmacology and Experimental Therapeutics Fast Forward* 308 2004; 838–845.

Mazur A, Maier JA, Rock E, Gueux E, Nowacki W and Rayssiguier Y. "Magnesium and the inflammatory response." 2006 April 19.

McAllister, Sean PhD. "THC and CBD enhances inhibitory effects on brain cancer." 2010 November 1.

Medical News Today. "Marijuana's active ingredient may slow progression of alzheimer's disease." 2006 October 1.
www.medicalnewstoday.com/releases/62616.php

Medical News Tody. "Parkinsons' helped by marijuana-lke chemicals in brain." 2007 February 11.
www.medicalnewstoday.com/releases/62616.php

Miller, Kelli. "Marijuana chemical may fight brain cancer." *WebMD Health News,* 2009 April 1.

National Institute on Aging. "About alzheimer's disease: alzheimer's basics."

National Organziation for the Reform of Marijuana Laws. "Cannabinoids reduce skin inflammation." 2007 June 14.

Nature 434. "Low dose cannabinoid therapy reduces progression of atherosclerosis in mice." 2005 April, 782–786.

Oyanaqi K. "The nature of the parkinsonism-dementia complex and amyotrophic lateral sclerosis of Guam and magnesium deficiency." *Neuropathology* Volume 26, 115–128.
www.ncbi.nlm.nih.gov/pubmed/15885623

Penner, Elizabeth A. MD, MPH et al. "The impact of marijuana use on glucose, insulin, and insulin resistance among us adults." *The American Journal of Medicine* 2013 July, Volume 126, Issue 7, Pages 583–589.

Reuters Health. "Cannabis may be helpful in Parkinson's disease." 2002 November 13.
www.cannabis-med.org/english/bulletin/ww_en_db_cannabis_artikel.php?id=131#2

Rubenowitz E, Axelsson G, Rylander R. "Magnesium and calcium in drinking water and death from acute myocardial infarction in women." *Epidemiology* 1999; 10:31–36.

Salazar, Maria. "Cannabinoid action induces autophagy-mediated cell death through stimiulation of ER stress in human glioma cells." *Journal of Clinical Investigation,* 2009;119(5) :1359–1372.

Sevick, J. Masek, K. "Role of cannabinoids in Parkinson's disease." Institute of Pharmacology, Academy of Sciences of the Czech Republic, Prague. *Drugs Aging* 2000 Jun; 16(6) : 391–5.

Ullrich, Oliver et al. "Brain's own cannabis compound protects against inflammation," *Neuron,* 2006 January 5.

Waseem, Muhammad, MD and Corden, Timothy E, MD. "Salicylate Toxicity," September 25, 2016.

Waseem, Muhammad, MD, MS. "Salicylate toxicity." *Medscape* 2016 September 25. http://emedicine.medscape.com/article/1009987-overview

Woolley, Pieta. "Vaccines show sinister side." *The Georgia Straight* 2006 March 23.

About the Author

Mark Sircus, Ac., OMD, DM (P), was trained in acupuncture and Asian medicine at the Institute of Traditional Medicine in Santa Fe and the School of Traditional Medicine of New England in Boston. He also served at the Central Public Hospital of Pochutla, Mexico. He is part of the Scientific Advisory and Research Development team of the Da Vinci College of Holistic Medicine. Dr. Sircus' articles have appeared in numerous journals and magazines throughout the world. In addition, he is the best-selling author of several books, including *Sodium Bicarbonate* and *Anti-Inflammatory Oxygen Therapy.*

Index

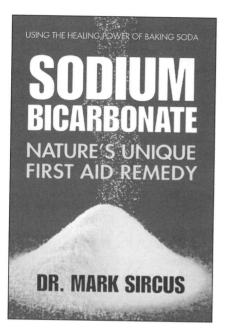

SODIUM BICARBONATE

Nature's Unique First Aid Remedy

Dr. Mark Sircus

What if there were a natural health-promoting substance that was inexpensive, available at any grocery store in the country, and probably sitting in your cupboard right now? There is. It is called sodium bicarbonate, although you may know it as baking soda. For years, sodium bicarbonate has been used on a daily basis as part of a number of hospital treatments, but most people remain unaware of its full therapeutic potential. In his new book, Dr. Mark Sircus shows how this common compound may be used in the alleviation, or possibly even prevention, of many forms of illness.

Sodium Bicarbonate begins with a basic overview of the everyday item known as baking soda, chronicling its long history of use as an effective home remedy. It then explains the role sodium bicarbonate plays in achieving optimal pH balance, which is revealed as an important factor in maintaining good health. The book goes on to detail how sodium bicarbonate and its effect on pH may benefit sufferers of a number of conditions, including kidney disease, fungal infection, influenza, hypertension, and even cancer. Finally, it lists the various ways in which sodium bicarbonate may be taken, suggesting the easiest and most effective method for your situation.

By providing a modern approach to this time-honored remedy, *Sodium Bicarbonate* illustrates the need to see baking soda in a whole new light. While it was once considered simply an ingredient in baked goods and toothpaste, sodium bicarbonate contains powerful properties that may help you balance your system, regain your wellbeing, and avoid future health problems.

$16.95 • 208 pages • 6 x 9-inch paperback • ISBN 978-0-7570-0394-3

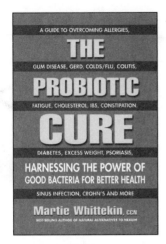

THE PROBIOTIC CURE

Harnessing the Power of Good Bacteria for Better Health

Martie Whittekin, CCN

Only recently have scientists recognized that an imbalance in the bacteria of your stomach can cause a host of serious disorders, from diabetes to ulcers. Now, best-selling health author Martie Whittekin has written *The Probiotic Cure,* a guide to overcoming many of our most common health issues.

Part One of *The Probiotic Cure* explains how our internal flora works to promote health and how it can become unbalanced due to a poor diet, medications, and other factors. It goes on to explain how this balance can be restored safely and effectively by using probiotics—good bacteria available in supplement form. Part Two discusses the most common health disorders that may arise from a bacterial imbalance and explains both conventional treatments and the probiotics approach to healing.

$16.95 • 176 pages • 6 x 9-inch paperback • ISBN 978-0-7570-0423-0

THE MAGNESIUM SOLUTION FOR HIGH BLOOD PRESSURE

How to Use Magnesium to Help Prevent & Relieve Hypertension Naturally

Jay S. Cohen, MD

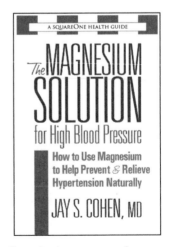

Approximately 50 percent of Americans have hypertension. Many medications are available to combat this condition, but they come with potential side effects. Fortunately, there is a remedy that's both safe and effective—magnesium. *The Magnesium Solution for High Blood Pressure* describes the best types of magnesium, explores appropriate dosage, and details the use of magnesium with hypertension meds.

$5.95 • 96 pages • 4 x 7-inch mass paperback • ISBN 978-0-7570-0255-7

ANTI-INFLAMMATORY OXYGEN THERAPY

Your Complete Guide to Understanding and Using Natural Oxygen Therapy

Dr. Mark Sircus

It is invisible, it is powerful, and it is life sustaining. It is oxygen. We inhale it every day of our lives, and while it makes up only 21 percent of the air we breathe, it is the key to our very existence. The more we learn about its healing properties, the more we recognize its tremendous potential as a medical treatment for many serious disorders. Yet few have known about its important therapeutic uses—until now. In *Anti-Inflammatory Oxygen*

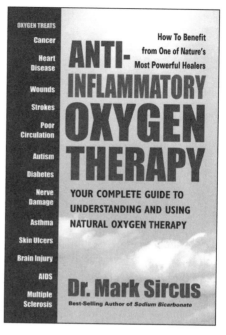

Therapy, best-selling author Dr. Mark Sircus examines the remarkable benefits oxygen therapy offers, from detoxification to treatments for a wide variety of disorders—from aging to gastric disorders to cancer.

While the term "oxygen therapy" conjures images of crucially ill patients lying in hospital beds with tubes strapped to their faces, this book will show that oxygen can offer so much more. Dr. Sircus first looks at the nature of oxygen and its purpose in the body. He then provides an understanding of how inflammation works to destroy the body's tissues over time, and how oxygen can reverse this process. He examines the current treatments that use hyperbaric oxygen chambers as well as newer protocols that employ this vital element. In addition, Dr. Sircus offers a simple, safe, and highly effective fifteen-minute technique that can be used in the privacy of your home so that you can enjoy maximum benefits for a healthier life.

If you are wondering why you haven't heard about this "miracle" treatment before, the fact is oxygen cannot be patented, it is not expensive, and you don't have to be a specialist to use it. Without a tremendous profit behind it, it's become a well-kept secret, but the facts speak for themselves. In this book, you will learn these life-altering facts—information that could change your health for the better.

$15.95 • 192 pages • 6 x 9-inch paperback • ISBN 978-0-7570-0415-5

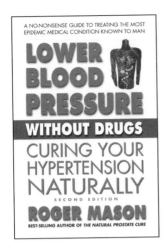

LOWER BLOOD PRESSURE WITHOUT DRUGS

SECOND EDITION

Curing Your Hypertension Naturally

Roger Mason

Over 65 million Americans have high blood pressure. Although prescription drugs may effectively treat this disorder, they can have dangerous side effects. Fortunately, natural alternatives are available.

In this updated edition of *Lower Blood Pressure Without Drugs,* best-selling author Roger Mason offers a nutritional approach to managing hypertension safely and naturally. First, you'll learn all about high blood pressure—what it is, what causes it, and how it is diagnosed. Then, you'll discover how a simple diet, rich in whole grains and low in fat, can improve both blood pressure and general health.

$9.95 • 128 pages • 6 x 9-inch paperback • ISBN 978-0-7570-0366-0

LOWER YOUR CHOLESTEROL WITHOUT DRUGS

SECOND EDITION

Curing High Cholesterol Naturally

Roger Mason

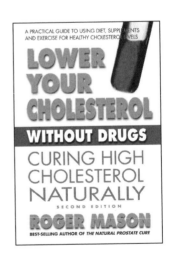

According to the American Heart Association, high cholesterol is the leading cause of coronary heart disease. While prescription drugs can lower cholesterol, they can also have undesired effects. But is a better option available?

In *Lower Your Cholesterol Without Drugs,* Roger Mason offers you a safe, effective way to treat this condition and improve your health. The book looks at the causes of high cholesterol and then explains how a balanced, vitamin-rich diet can lower cholesterol while enhancing your well-being. Information is also provided on natural supplements that can help lower even genetically high cholesterol.

$9.95 • 128 pages • 6 x 9-inch paperback • ISBN 978-0-7570-0367-7

YOUR BLOOD NEVER LIES

How to Read a Blood Test for a Longer, Healthier Life

James B. LaValle, RPh, CCN

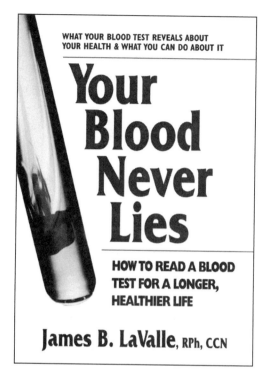

If you're like most people, you probably rely on your doctor to interpret the results of your blood tests, which contain a wealth of information on the state of your health. A blood test can tell you how well your liver and kidneys are functioning, your potential for heart disease and diabetes, the strength of your immune system, the chemical profile of your blood, and many other important facts about the state of your health. And yet, most of us cannot decipher these results ourselves, nor can we even formulate the right questions to ask about them—or we couldn't, until now.

In *Your Blood Never Lies,* best-selling author Dr. James LaValle clears the mystery surrounding blood test results. In simple language, he explains all the information found on a typical lab report—the medical terminology, the numbers and percentages, and the laboratory jargon—and makes it accessible. This means that you will be able to look at your own blood test results and understand the significance of each biological marker being measured. To help you take charge of your health, Dr. LaValle also recommends the most effective standard and complementary treatments for dealing with any problematic findings. Rounding out the book are explanations of lab values that do not appear on the standard blood test, but that should be requested for a more complete picture of your current physiological condition.

A blood test can reveal so much about your body, but only if you can interpret the results. *Your Blood Never Lies* provides the up-to-date information you need to understand your results and take control of your life.

$16.95 • 368 pages • 6 x 9-inch paperback • ISBN 978-0-7570-0350-9

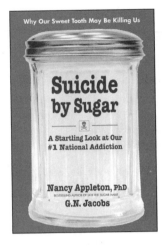

SUICIDE BY SUGAR

A Startling Look at Our #1 National Addiction

Nancy Appleton, PhD, and G.N. Jacobs

More than two decades ago, Nancy Appleton's *Lick the Sugar Habit* exposed the health dangers of America's high-sugar diet. Now, in *Suicide by Sugar*, Appleton, along with journalist G.N. Jacobs, presents a broader view of the problems caused by our favorite ingredient.

The authors offer startling facts that link a range of disorders—from dementia and hypoglycemia to obesity and cancer—to our growing addiction to sugar. Rounding out the book is a sound diet plan along with a number of recipes for sweet, easy-to-prepare delectable dishes, all made without sugar or fruit.

$15.95 • 192 pages • 6 x 9-inch paperback • ISBN 978-0-7570-0306-6

HEALTH AT GUNPOINT

The FDA's Silent War Against Health Freedom

James J. Gormley

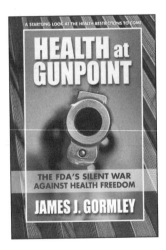

While the original intent of the Food and Drug Administration may have been honorable, over time, unfortunately, the mission has become tainted by lobbyists. *Health at Gunpoint* presents a history of the agency's long battle against health products and examines some of its most controversial decisions.

Now, the FDA is again poised to make decisions that would have a major impact on the public, this time, by imposing restrictions that could eliminate many of the nutritional supplements we take. *Health at Gunpoint* not only sheds light on what is happening, but also prepares us for the coming battle.

$14.95 • 176 pages • 6 x 9-inch paperback • ISBN 978-0-7570-0381-3